The Pocket Guide
to Health Promotion

The Pocket Guide
to Health Promotion

Glenn Laverack

Mc
Graw
Hill
Education Open University Press

Open University Press
McGraw-Hill Education
McGraw-Hill House
Shoppenhangers Road
Maidenhead
Berkshire
England
SL6 2QL

email: enquiries@openup.co.uk
world wide web: www.openup.co.uk

and Two Penn Plaza, New York, NY 10121-2289, USA

First published 2014

A catalogue record of this book is available from the British Library

ISBN-13: 978-0-335-26472-8
ISBN-10: 0-335-26472-7
eISBN: 978-0-335-26473-5

Library of Congress Cataloging-in-Publication Data
CIP data applied for

Fictitious names of companies, products, people, characters and/or data that may
be used herein (in case studies or in examples) are not intended to represent
any real individual, company, product or event.

Printed and bound by CPI Group (UK) Ltd, Croydon, CR0 4YY

*I would like to thank James Woodall,
David Pattison and Laura Aaben for their
invaluable comments on the draft book.*

*To Elizabeth, Ben, Holly and Rebecca just
because I love them.*

Contents

List of tables

List of figures

Introduction

The 'Pocket Guide to Health Promotion' has been written to be an invaluable companion for practitioners, students and anyone who is passionate about promoting health. Most of all, it has been written for field workers who every day strive to deliver health promotion programmes, sometimes without adequate support or resources, to the best of their ability. The idea for the pocket guide came from my own experiences with international field workers and their need for a book that covered only the most essential aspects of health promotion in practice.

The 'Pocket Guide to Health Promotion' is not intended to be a theoretical foundation or a manual of how to implement specific interventions. The purpose is to provide clear practice pathways within an empowerment framework for health promotion. I therefore intentionally do not include approaches that depend heavily on information transfer and behaviour change such as health education and social marketing. A key question that is commonly asked by field workers is: Do we want to help others to empower themselves or to simply change their behaviour? This is an important ethical and practical issue that is addressed in the pocket guide.

The pocket guide is divided into three parts

The pocket guide is divided into three parts that together cover the key stages of a programme cycle: management, planning, strategy selection, strategy implementation and evaluation.

Part I of the pocket guide (health promotion explained) covers chapters 1 to 3 and explains the importance of enabling people to gain more control over their lives and health. Chapter 1 explains the interpretation of health promotion and the ways it can be usefully viewed, as a community-based, bottom-up practice within a political context. Chapter 2 provides five entries that are listed in alphabetical order of the key concepts central to health promotion: advocacy, determinants of health, empowerment, power and salutogenesis. Chapter 3 provides five entries that are listed in alphabetical order of the key methods central to health promotion: asset-based community development, harm reduction, innovative communication technologies, lobbying and moral suasion. Each entry has been included because it can help field workers to better implement empowerment approaches in health promotion programmes. Further information for each entry is provided as key texts to encourage the reader to gain a more in-depth understanding of the subject.

Online resources such as manuals of how to implement specific interventions have not been included in this pocket guide because these are regularly changed and would not be useful to the content of the pocket guide.

Part II of the pocket guide (health promotion programmes) covers chapters 4 to 10 and discusses the programme cycle approach to health promotion: management, planning, strategy selection, strategy implementation and evaluation. Chapter 4 begins with a discussion of how best to manage the programme cycle, including leadership skills, conflict resolution and using an ethical approach. Chapter 5 explains the planning process, including important issues in the design such as the programme time frame and size, setting realistic objectives and the central role of needs assessment. Chapter 6 discusses strategy selection, the 'art and science' of health promotion and the use of theory, strategic approaches and a settings approach. Chapter 7, strategy implementation, explains effective approaches, methods and tools for individuals and groups. Chapter 8, strategy implementation, explains effective approaches, methods and tools for communities. Chapter 9 focuses on the policy process and how practitioners can work with other partners – for example, through pressure groups and social movements – to influence change. Chapter 10 discusses how health promotion practice can be evaluated and the use of different methods that can promote the participation and empowerment of others.

Part III of the pocket guide provides a glossary of terms, a full list of references and an index to assist ease of access to further information for the reader's own interests.

How to use the 'Pocket Guide to Health Promotion'

The pocket guide is a convenient source book for the understanding of key concepts and methods used in health promotion. The guide does not have to be read sequentially. Instead, the reader can simply access any chapter, entry or combination of headings to gain easy access. The reader can quickly access the information that they require, aided by practical examples and insightful remarks provided in the text. The rationale for the choice of headings is intended to help the reader to better understand how health promotion theory can be applied in practice.

In this pocket guide I have purposefully chosen the term 'programme' to cover the different types of delivery of health promotion projects, interventions and activities. I have also used the term 'partners' to cover the different stakeholders, beneficiaries and target audiences in health promotion programmes.

It is recommended that the reader firstly chooses a heading listed in the contents, or in the index of the pocket guide, that matches the information about which they wish to gain a better understanding. Alternatively, in chapter 2 (five useful concepts in health promotion) and chapter 3 (five useful methods in health promotion) the reader can choose a specific entry. Each entry has been written to provide the reader with a precise definition along with a theoretical and, where appropriate, a historical background. For entries with a practical purpose, examples of application in a programme context have also been provided. If the reader requires further information they can use one of the key texts listed at the end of the entry.

This pocket guide has been written to inspire the field workers of health promotion. These people work at the 'cutting edge' of practice, often alone and with limited support but they are committed to enabling others to improve their lives and health.

PART I
Health promotion explained

1 Health promotion in context

Health promotion is a contested concept partly because its broad range of activities overlap with other professional fields including health education and public health. The interpretation of health promotion has evolved historically and the different approaches that it uses have developed without any one remaining dominant. This evolution is represented in the series of World Health Organization charters and statements (see box 1.1) and by various theories and approaches (see chapter 6).

Health promotion defined

Health promotion can be broadly viewed as a set of principles involving equity and empowerment and as a practice that encompasses a range of communication, capacity-building and politically orientated activities. The goal is to enable others to gain more control over the influences on their lives and to improve their health (Laverack, 2007).

Two key World Health Organization charters that have helped define health promotion are the Ottawa Charter (WHO, 1986) and the Bangkok Charter for Health Promotion in a Globalized World (WHO, 2005). The definition provided in the Ottawa Charter is still the most commonly used and universally recognised but has not been updated in over 25 years even though health promotion practice has changed. For example, the role of the determinants of health (see chapter 2) has arisen as a new area of professional concern in health promotion through the work of the Commission on Social Determinants of Health (WHO, 2008). The development and use of innovative new technologies (see chapter 3) in health promotion have also changed the way in which practitioners communicate and engage with individuals and communities.

The Ottawa Charter is still the most commonly used and universally recognised definition by practitioners: 'Health promotion is the process of enabling people to increase control over, and to improve, their health' (WHO, 1986: 1).

The Bangkok Charter defines health promotion as being 'the process of enabling people to increase control over their health and its determinants, and thereby improve their health' (WHO, 2005: 2), a clear endorsement that health promotion has an important role in improving health through influencing its determinants. However, unlike the Ottawa Charter, the Bangkok Charter does not provide a framework that practitioners can use in their day-to day work. The Bangkok Charter is intended for a different audience: governments and politicians at all levels, the private sector, international organisations and civil society. The commitments of the Bangkok Charter are to make the promotion of health central to the global development agenda and a core responsibility for the whole of government and for corporate practice. These commitments require strong intergovernmental and corporate agreements for action, which is perhaps why the Bangkok Charter has never achieved the same level of patronage and support as has the more practice-based Ottawa Charter.

Experience has shown that the influence of a health promotion charter has a much better chance of success when it is backed by a movement of both professionals and civil society.

Declarations and statements of health promotion

The global direction and leadership that has helped to shape the way we view health promotion has been marked by key World Health Organization declarations and statements that define and legitimise new approaches in both theory and practice. In particular, the following charters and statements have made a contribution:

- The 1986 Ottawa Charter
- The 1988 Adelaide Conference Statement
- The 1991 Sunsdvall Conference Statement
- The 1997 Jakarta Conference Statement
- The 2000 Mexico Global Conference Statement
- The 2005 Bangkok Charter for Health Promotion in a Globalized World
- The 2009 Nairobi Global Conference Statement
- The 2013 Helsinki Global Conference on Health Promotion Statement.

Health promotion and public health

Public health is an approach that aims to promote health, to prevent disease, to treat illnesses, to prolong life, to care for the infirm and to provide

Box 1.1 Key WHO charters and statements

The 1986 Ottawa Charter for Health Promotion (WHO, 1986)

The first international conference and a response to growing expectations for a new public health movement. The conference statement defined health promotion as 'the process of enabling people to increase control over, and to improve, their health. Not just the responsibility of the health sector, but . . . beyond healthy lifestyles to wellbeing' (WHO, 1986: 1). The conference identified a number of prerequisites or fundamental conditions and resources, and expanded the outcomes for health promotion beyond the absence of disease or the adoption of healthy lifestyles. The Charter defined five health promotion action areas for achieving better health:

1　Building healthy public policy
2　Creating supportive environments
3　Strengthening community action
4　Developing personal skills
5　Re-orienting health services.

It also described three important roles for health promoters: advocating, enabling and mediating. The Ottawa Charter set a new standard and became the founding document of the 'new' health promotion movement.

The 1988 Adelaide Conference Statement (WHO, 1988)

Addressed the first of the five action areas from the Ottawa Charter: building healthy public policy. The conference statement stated that 'health is both a fundamental human right and a sound social investment'. It took the discussion on the link between inequalities in health and public policy further than before in the context of health promotion.

The 1991 Sunsdvall Conference Statement (WHO, 1991)

The first WHO health promotion conference to have a global perspective, this addressed the second of the five action areas from the Ottawa Charter: creating supportive environments. The term 'supportive environments' refers to the protection of people from threats to health, and to enabling people to expand their capabilities and develop self-reliance in health. They encompass

(continued)

where people live, their local community, their home, and where they work and play, including people's access to resources for health and opportunities for empowerment. Action to create supportive environments for health has many dimensions, and may include direct political action to develop and implement policies and regulations which help create supportive environments, and economic action, particularly in relation to fostering sustainable economic development and social action.

The 1997 Jakarta Conference Statement (WHO, 1997)

This statement endorsed health as a basic human right, affirmed the five action areas of the Ottawa Charter and proposed (somewhat controversially) that new partnerships, especially with the private sector, were important to the success of health promotion. The conference also affirmed that comprehensive approaches to health promotion such as the settings approach offer practical opportunities for the implementation of strategies.

The 2000 Mexico Global Conference for Health Promotion (WHO, 2000)

Sought to demonstrate how health promotion strategies add value to the effectiveness of health and development policies, programmes and projects, particularly those that aim to improve the health and quality of life of people living in adverse circumstances. The conference statement recognised that health is not only an outcome of, but also an important input into, economic development and equity.

The 2005 Bangkok Charter for Health Promotion in a Globalized World (WHO, 2005)

Seen as the first attempt to revise the Ottawa Charter, the Bangkok Charter identified actions, commitments and pledges required to address the determinants of health in a globalised world through health promotion. It extended the definition of health promotion to also address the determinants of health: 'the process of enabling people to increase control over their health and its determinants, and thereby improve their health. It is a core function of public health and contributes to the work of tackling communicable and non-communicable diseases and other threats to health' (WHO, 2005: 2).

(continued)

| The 2009 Nairobi Global Conference on Health Promotion (WHO, 2009) | The call to action identifies key strategies and commitments urgently required for closing the implementation gap in health and development through health promotion. The main strategies are presented under five sub-themes: building capacity or health promotion, strengthening health systems, partnerships and inter-sectoral action, community empowerment, and health literacy and health behaviours. A plan of action is still required with clearly defined roles, responsibilities and timelines for the implementation and follow-up of the conference statement. |
| The 2013 Helsinki Global Conference on Health Promotion (WHO, 2013) | Facilitated the exchange of experiences and lessons learnt for implementing the Health in All Policies (HiAP) approach. The conference provided guidance, especially to member states, on what HiAP is, why it is important and how to implement it in the future. A Health in All Policies approach considers health impacts across all sectors such as agriculture, education, the environment, housing and transport, to achieve better health outcomes. It complements a Whole of Government (WoG) approach, which focuses on public coherence, coordination and efficiency. |

health services. Traditionally, such goals have been used to curb the spread of infectious diseases and to protect the wellbeing of the general population, whilst others see a much greater role in regulation and reducing inequalities in health (Baggott, 2010). Public health and health promotion activities do overlap, particularly in the areas of improvement and prevention. However, public health is a much broader concept that covers a number of specialist areas including treatment, diagnosis and health service provision. Public health professionals may therefore call themselves 'health promoters' or 'health communicators', whilst many more who look to this concept for models, professional legitimacy and resource occupy jobs such as health visitors and environmental health officers.

The most practical way forward is to view health promotion as encompassing a range of educational, skills development and community development activities that are part of a broader public health framework.

Health promotion and health education

The debate about the overlap between health promotion and health education began in the 1980s when the range of activities involved in promoting health widened to overcome the narrow focus on lifestyle and behavioural approaches. These activities involved more than just the giving of information and aimed for strategies that achieved political action and social mobilisation. The emphasis on individual responsibility in health education also led to accusations of 'victim-blaming', making people feel guilty about their poor state of health even though certain risk factors were outside of their control: for example, being made unemployed.

Whilst there is no universally accepted definition of health education the term is traditionally regarded to represent planned opportunities for people to learn about health and to make changes to their behaviour (Naidoo and Wills, 2009). Health education provides the latest technical information, motivating people to change unhealthy behaviours by giving them the confidence to make those changes.

The role of the health educator is to design and implement learning activities, and to provide training, instruction and skills development. The guiding principle of health education is to facilitate people to make informed choices about their health behaviours.

Health education is often assumed to be the first step towards awareness-raising and changing attitudes following which the individual then volunteers to change their behaviour.

Tones and Tilford (2001) have suggested that health education and health promotion have a symbiotic relationship. Health education provides the agenda setting and aspects of critical education in health promotion. But, whereas health education is aimed at informing people to influence their future decision-making, health promotion aims at complementary social and political actions (Green and Kreuter, 2004). Health education around obesity in adolescents, for example, might include school-based awareness-raising programmes or exercise classes. Health promotion would include this but also extend further to legislation on food advertising and restricting access to unhealthy products in school shops and canteens (Laverack, 2004). Health education alone therefore is seen as being insufficient to achieve positive health outcomes or to influence the broader structural causes of powerlessness.

The most practical way forward is to view health promotion as including a range of educational and skills development activities that can be called 'health education'.

Health promotion and the political context

Health promotion is, or should be, a political activity, as many of its actions have political consequences for those in society, for example, through health legislation and policy. To be more politically effective, practitioners must fully understand the sources of their own power and how this can be used to help others to have a greater influence on the political context.

> Rudolf Virchow, a 19th-century health reformer, made no distinction between being a health professional and a political activist. To Virchow all disease had two causes, one pathological and the other political.

People have traditionally expressed their discontent through, for example, signing a petition or writing a letter to lobby someone in a position of authority. However, those who are poor are often unsuccessful in using these types of indirect strategies because they lack the resources and leverage necessary to have an influence. People that are able to persuade others in authority to make changes do so by using direct tactics such as legal action or mass protests as a means to inform politicians and policymakers about their grievances. The purpose is to shift political opinion about a particular decision, especially when it favours one group's interests or has not yet arrived at a firm view on an issue.

Economic conditions in many countries have given rise to governments introducing public policies that reduce social and economic structures, deregulate labour and financial markets, and stimulate commerce and investment (Navarro, 2009). For everyday living conditions this can mean cutting pay and jobs, freezing benefits and welfare payments, and reducing opportunities for self-determination (Nathanson and Hopper, 2010). Civil society resistance is especially important when governments are pursuing a tighter agenda and practitioners can facilitate others to engage in different forms of political activity. Practitioners also have the right of exercising their own voices as individuals – for example, through their participation in advocacy groups that support the actions of others who they believe suffer from an inequality. Professional associations can also endorse the concerns of others to legitimise their cause – for example, the support of the medical profession to Action on Smoking and Health (ASH). The credibility that the support has given to this advocacy group has contributed to a nationwide ban on smoking in public places in some European countries because of the associated health risks of passive smoking (ASH, 2012).

Health promotion and the bureaucratic context

Health promotion often operates within bureaucratic settings such as government departments and institutions consisting of a number of distinctive positions of authority with specialist duties that are formally defined. Professionally positioning oneself within the hierarchy of a bureaucratic setting also provides some degree of legitimacy and status. If it is true that health promotion is largely a bureaucratic activity then it is also true that some organisations remain committed to ways of thinking and acting that can inhibit empowering approaches. Despite the intent to empower others, health promotion organisations and their staff may retain control over the activities that they deliver rather than relinquish responsibility to their partners. If a programme, for example, does not provide the opportunity for its partners to identify their own needs, then this further enables paternalistic approaches to be used (Braunack-Mayer and Louise, 2008). This allows greater control by the practitioner who selects the issues to be addressed and the approaches to be used for management, implementation and evaluation.

Health promotion programmes can sometimes operate within a contradiction: practitioners continued to exert control over their partners whilst at the same time using an empowering discourse.

To avoid a contradiction between discourse and practice in health promotion the programme design must ensure that all the partners are fully involved in the planning, implementation and evaluation of its activities. This can include a local needs assessment (chapter 5), appropriate strategy selection (chapter 6) and strategy implementation (chapters 7 and 8). It can also include the engagement and support of other sectors to deliver health and equity outcomes in a Whole of Government approach.

Health in All Policies

Many governments have a dedicated health promotion workforce but the main human resource is to be found in other sectors – for example, in education, social welfare and transport. A Whole of Government (WoG) approach focuses on public coherence, coordination and efficiency. When a health issue is not a WoG priority, then a Health in All Policies (HiAP) approach can be used to engage and support other sectors to deliver the desired health and equity outcomes. HiAP is an approach which emphasises that wellbeing is largely influenced by government sectors other than health and highlights the interactions between different policies. By considering health impacts across all policies such as agriculture, education, the environment, housing and transport, health outcomes can be better achieved. A HiAP approach improves the accountability of policymakers for health impacts and includes an emphasis on the consequences of public policies on health systems, determinants of health and wellbeing (WHO, 2014).

Health promotion has an important leadership role in HiAP to support other sectors to achieve their goals in a way which can improve health and wellbeing.

The role of the health promotion practitioner

Health promotion practice is set within a programme design, often directed by an outside agency or practitioner. The programme addresses prioritised needs that are reflected in its goals, identifying in advance suitable indicators of progress and the assessment of risks. Practitioners are employed to deliver information, resources and services and to manage the programme. Practitioners call themselves 'health promoters' or 'public health workers' whilst many more who look to the role of health promotion are nurses, teachers and doctors. The term 'partners' covers the range of people who act as the recipients of the information, resources and services being delivered to promote health: for example, pregnant women, school children, the unemployed, consumer or patient groups and community-based organisations that have been formed to address a specific health-related issue (Laverack, 2009).

A major role of the practitioner has been concerned with education, training and specialist services – for example, that of a nurse providing advice about self-treatment to her patient. This role has helped to broaden the image of the practitioner as a health professional with 'expert' power and with access to superior technical resources, skills and knowledge. Practitioners can and often do play an important role in facilitating change in programme partners, either on a one-to-one basis or through working with groups and communities. Practitioners who are in a position of relative power can work to enable their partners, who are often in a relatively powerless position, by providing information and resources and by using their professional influence to legitimise the concerns of others.

> The role of the practitioner is that of an 'enabler', gaining the trust
> of and establishing common ground with others, to help them to
> empower themselves.

Empowerment or behaviour change?

The difference between delivering an empowering approach compared
to delivering a behaviour change approach is in the selection of the
strategies used in a programme. If the strategy gives the practitioner
the authority to control the situation – for example, through setting the
agenda or releasing specific resources – it is less likely to be empowering. If it facilitates a process of needs assessment, planning and capacity-
building towards political action by the programme partners, it has a
much better chance of being empowering.

> In a professional context the key question is: Do I want to help others
> to empower themselves or to simply change their behaviour?

Both the behaviour change and the empowerment approaches are
used to achieve health promotion goals. Per-Anders Tengland (2013), a
health philosopher, identifies that the behaviour change approach has
several moral problems. First of all, it is overly paternalistic and often
disregards the individual's own perception of what is important. Fur-
thermore, the behaviour change approach can lead to 'victim blaming'
and stigmatisation, and to increased inequalities in health, as its focus
is on individual behaviours instead of the 'causes of the causes' of poor
health. The empowerment approach does not have these problems but
can lead to empowering some groups more than others; the focus is not
primarily on health and empowered people might still choose to behave
in ways that risk damaging their health. However, he argues that the
empowerment approach, on the whole, is superior to the behaviour
change approach.

Both approaches aim to achieve improvements in health. However,
the additional advantage of empowerment is that it strengthens the
whole individual, group or community, – their autonomy, skills, and
general control – in achieving better, healthier and more sustainable
lives. Behaviour changes do sometimes lead to the development of the
ability for autonomy and control, but, if they do, this is usually as a secondary effect, such as a feeling of greater self-esteem following weight
loss. The solution, therefore, should not simply be behaviour change,

but the attainment of more autonomous choice and empowerment. Solely targeting behaviour change seldom addresses more important issues such as powerlessness or inequity. For some people, health is also secondary to other personal goals in their lives and they may be willing to risk their health in order to pursue these goals. This is not compatible with the assumptions of the behaviour change approach but it can be accommodated within an empowerment approach.

Key points of the chapter

- Health promotion is a contested concept but there are established approaches that can guide both theory and practice.
- Empowerment and political activity are central to health promotion practice.
- Health promotion practice should avoid the contradiction of using an empowering discourse whilst at the same time using a controlling practice.
- Health promotion can be viewed as encompassing a range of educational and skills development activities that can be called 'health education'.
- Health promotion can be viewed as encompassing a range of educational, skills and community development activities that are part of a broader public health framework.
- The empowerment approach, on the whole, is morally superior to the behaviour change approach.

2 | Five useful concepts in health promotion

In this chapter I explore five key concepts central to health promotion: advocacy, determinants of health, empowerment, power and salutogenesis. Each concept is listed with a precise definition along with a theoretical and, where appropriate, a historical background. For entries with a practical purpose, examples of application in a programme context have also been provided. For further information, key texts have been listed at the end of the entry.

Advocacy

Advocacy involves people acting on behalf of themselves or on behalf of others to argue a position and to influence the outcome of decisions. In health promotion, advocacy initiatives are usually started to support particular causes, interest groups and ideologies (Smithies and Webster, 1998).

Some of the key forms of advocacy are listed below.

- Health advocacy supports and promotes healthcare rights as well as enhancing community health and policy initiatives: for example, the availability, safety and quality of care. It focuses on education and relies on expert knowledge rather than inserting lay knowledge into expert systems.
- Media advocacy is the strategic use of the mass media as a resource to advance a policy initiative and aims to influence the selection, framing and debate of specific topics. The goal of media advocacy is to target the ways in which issues come to be regarded as newsworthy, to help set the debate and to frame the problem and the solution in an appropriate way so that others can understand the issue (Wallack et al., 1993).
- Collective or mass advocacy occurs when groups and organisations campaign on issues that are important to their members and who then speak out for themselves or influence what others say in a campaign (Loue et al., 2003).
- Peer advocacy occurs when a person agrees to act on behalf of another: for example, volunteers who are recruited to act on behalf of service users at a Citizens' Advice Bureau.

- Self-advocacy occurs when individuals or groups share the same concerns or act on their own behalf.
- Legal advocacy occurs when a legally qualified person is employed to act on behalf of others as an advocate, solicitor or barrister (Smithies and Webster, 1998).

In practice, the different forms of advocacy can overlap: for example, self-advocacy groups can play an important role in supporting peer advocacy and collective advocacy can support the efforts of self-advocacy groups.

Action on Smoking and Health (ASH) is the name of a number of autonomous advocacy groups throughout the world that have been successful in taking action against the risks associated with tobacco smoking. ASH uses a dual approach of information and networking, and advocacy and campaigning. ASH has had some success: for example, in 2007 it won its campaign for a ban on smoking in enclosed public places in England including bars and private members clubs, as well as cafés, restaurants and workplaces (ASH, 2012). ASH purposefully uses unthreatening strategies such as advocacy because its charitable status creates a dependence on government funding. Advocacy does not therefore always challenge those in authority to force them to make the system more equitable.

Health promotion should do more than helping others to speak on their own behalf, and should go beyond advocacy to enable others to take more control of their lives. This can be achieved through more direct actions to force social and political change including legal action, protests, lobbying and consumer boycotts (Labonte and Laverack, 2008).

Key texts

Loue, S., Lloyd, L. S. and O'Shea, D. J. (2003) *Community health advocacy*. New York: Kluwer Academic/Plenum.

Lustig, S. (2012) *Advocacy strategies for health and mental health professionals. From patients to policies*. New York: Springer.

Young, L. and Everitt, J. (2004) *Advocacy groups*. Vancouver, BC: The University of British Columbia Press.

Determinants of health

The determinants of health encompass the economic and social conditions that influence the health of individuals, communities and populations. Addressing the determinants of health requires an approach that recognises that health is influenced by how societies themselves are structured (Mouy and Barr, 2006), a long-term approach to change the causes of social and economic inequality including unemployment and poor education services.

The social determinants of health

The social determinants of health are the conditions in which people are born, grow, live, work and age, circumstances that are shaped by the distribution of power and resources and which are themselves influenced by policy choices (WHO, 2008).

The social gradient: Life expectancy is shorter for people further down the social ladder and who are likely to experience more disease and ill health than those nearer the top in society.

Stress: People that are worried, anxious and unable to cope, psychologically, suffer from stress that over long periods of time can damage their health, through, for example, high blood pressure, stroke and depression.

Early life: Slow physical growth and poor emotional support can result in a lifetime of poor health and a reduced psychological functioning in adulthood. Poor fetal development – linked to, for example, stress, addiction and poor prenatal care – is a risk for health in later life.

Social exclusion: Poverty, discrimination and racism can all contribute to social exclusion. These processes prevent people from participating in health and education services, are psychologically damaging and can lead to illness and premature death.

Work: Whilst having a job is generally healthier than not having a job, stress in the workplace increases the risk of ill health: for example, through mental illness.

Unemployment: Job security increases health; unemployment, or the insecurity of losing one's job, causes more illness and premature death. The health effects of unemployment are linked to psychological factors such as anxiety that can be brought on by problems of debt.

Social support: Having friends, good social relationships and supportive networks can improve health. People have better health when they feel cared for, loved, esteemed and valued. Conversely, people who do not have these factors in their lives suffer from poorer health and premature death.

Addiction: Alcohol dependence, illicit drug use and smoking are not only markers of social and economic disadvantage but are also important factors in worsening health. People can enter into addictive relationships to provide a temporary release from the harsh social and economic conditions in which they live, but as a result their long-term health can be damaged.

Food: A good diet and an adequate supply of food are important to health and wellbeing. A poor diet can cause malnutrition or obesity and can contribute to, for example, cancer and diabetes, and is often associated with people who are lower on the social gradient.

Transport: The reliance on mechanised transport has resulted in people taking less exercise, along with an increase in fatal road accidents and more pollution. Other forms of transport such as cycling and walking increase exercise levels and help people to reduce obesity and diseases such as diabetes and strokes (Wilkinson, 2003).

Within countries, the lower an individual's socio-economic status and position on the social gradient, the worse is their health.

Social injustice and health inequities manifest across civil society and reflect unequal differences in the wealth and power of people. Serious efforts to reduce social injustice and health inequities involve changing the distribution of power within society, empowering people to address their needs and, in so doing, to change the unfair distribution of social and material resources. Governments can therefore have a significant impact on the social determinants of health through the policies and legislation that they authorise, by, among other things:

- improving the standards of teaching and resource allocation to schools;
- ensuring a minimum wage and regulated working hours;
- creating better opportunities to find work;
- protecting vulnerable and marginalised groups;
- providing preventive services and parental education about child care;
- creating better access to affordable child care facilities;
- building community support and social interaction;
- improving access to public transport; and
- improving access to public exercise facilities such as cycle paths (Wilkinson, 2003).

Key texts

Cannon, M. and Perkins, J. (2009) *Social justice handbook*. Nottingham: IVP Books.

Marmot, M. and Wilkinson, R. (eds) (2009) *Social determinants of health*. Oxford: Oxford University Press.

World Health Organization (2008) *Closing the gap in a generation. Commission on Social Determinants of Health. Final Report*. Geneva: World Health Organization.

Empowerment

Empowerment in the broadest sense is a process by which people who perceive themselves as being disadvantaged work together to increase control over events that influence their lives (Werner, 1988).

Despite the year of the above definition, it reflects how others have subsequently given the term a similarly positive value, largely developed in western value systems and placing a strong emphasis on individual and community responsibility. It also embodies the notion that empowerment must come from within an individual, group or community and cannot be given to them.

It is through the process of community empowerment that people are best able to achieve the broader social and political change that is necessary to address the inequalities that influence their lives. Social change refers to societal norms, beliefs and behaviours that have an influence on others: for example, making smoking around others (resulting in passive smoking) an anti-social behaviour. Political change refers to policy, legislation and governance that have a direct influence on others: for example, policy prohibiting smoking in public places. Community empowerment is also an outcome that can include the redistribution of resources, a decrease in powerlessness or success in achieving social and political change. But it is as a process that it is most consistently used in practice, one that promotes the participation of people, organisations and communities towards increased individual and collective control. As a process, community empowerment is best considered as a continuum representing progressively more organised and broadly based forms of collective action. The groups and organisations that develop have their own dynamics; they may flourish for a time then fade away, for reasons as much to do with changes in the community as with a lack of broader political or financial support. This offers a simple, linear interpretation of what can be a more fluid and complex process. Nonetheless, the concept of a continuum provides a valuable tool to help practitioners to understand how they can become involved in empowering approaches (Laverack, 2004).

People with the ability to control decisions at the political and economic level constrain the ability of other people to exercise choice at the individual level.

Gaining influence on economic, political and social change will inevitably involve a struggle with those already holding power. Working in empowering ways is therefore a political activity because it challenges the structures of bureaucracy and authority that can sometimes create inequity and social injustice. The role of health promotion is to enable others to challenge the causes of their powerlessness, such as inequitable policy. How this can be best achieved is discussed in detail in chapters 7, 8 and 9.

Key texts

Kendall, S. (ed.) (1998) *Health and empowerment: Research and practice.* London: Arnold.

Laverack, G. (2007) *Health promotion practice: Building empowered communities.* Maidenhead: Open University Press.

Wallerstein, N. (2006) *What is the evidence on effectiveness of empowerment to improve health?* (Health Evidence Network report) Copenhagen: WHO Regional Office for Europe.

Power

Power is commonly interpreted as the capacity of some to produce intended and foreseen effects on others, even against their will (Wrong, 1988). One person, group or organisation then has influence and mastery over others.

Zero-sum power creates a 'win/lose' situation. My power over you, plus your absence of that power, equals zero (thus the term, 'zero-sum'). I win and you lose. For you to gain power, you must seize it from me. If you can, you win and I lose. It is important to understand that power has to be gained or seized by those who want to achieve it, by raising the position of one person or group, whilst simultaneously lowering it for another person or group (Laverack, 2004). The role of health promotion is to assist some to gain power, control over resources or decision-making, over others, and this can become a difficult issue. David Zakus and Catherine Lysack (1998), two Canadian health researchers, argue that health promotion practice that works from a zero-sum construction of power actually increases unhealthy competition between people and decreases healthy community capacity and cohesion. They suggest that by empowering some at the expense of others in a zero-sum situation, health promoters are helping to break down the ties that hold a community together. However, communities are not homogeneous and already consist of competing heterogeneous individuals and groups. Health promoters cannot therefore avoid empowering some whilst not others through the programmes that they deliver. However, this issue can become a problem if the target group is unpopular, such as people engaging in drug use, or if the strategy used is unpopular with government, such as harm reduction.

There is another important use of power, a 'non-zero-sum' form, that is 'win/win', since it is based on the idea that if any one person or group gains, everyone else gains. Knowledge, trust, caring and other aspects of our social relationships with one another are examples of non-zero-sum power. Perhaps unsurprisingly, health promoters often gravitate towards the non-zero-sum formulation. Certainly, much of the discourse of health promotion emphasising participation, caring and responsibility to others addresses the exercise of power in which all people can benefit. Power is no longer seen as a commodity, such as wealth, or as the comparative status and authority that this might confer. Rather, the non-zero-sum takes the form of relationship behaviours based on respect, generosity, service to others, a free flow of information and the commitment to the ethics of caring and justice. The role of the health promoter in this construction of power is to use these attributes to engender them in others – for example, through mentoring and counselling.

In practice, health promotion simultaneously involves zero-sum and non-zero-sum formulations of power. Power cannot be given but communities can be enabled by health promoters to take more control by identifying their own power base (access to resources and influence) and then understanding how this can be acted upon to enable others.

To better understand how power is exercised either positively (the sharing of control with others) or negatively (the use of control to exert influence over others against their will) within health promotion, it is helpful to consider three of its simplest forms: 'power-from-within' 'power-over' and 'power-with'.

Power-from-within

Power-from-within can be described as an experience of self, a personal or psychological power and gaining (a sense of) control over one's life (Rissel, 1994). The goal of power-from-within is to increase feelings of value and a sense of individual mastery and to increase the notion of self, without access to or control over resources. Individuals can therefore gain power-from-within without necessarily having to accumulate power as money, or status or authority. Feminist theory, for example, holds that even in the most male-dominated societies women have power, their power-from-within, and can therefore both have and lack power at the same time in society.

Power-over

Power-over describes social relationships in which one party is made to do what another party wishes them to, despite their resistance and even if it may not be in their best interests (Wrong, 1988). The exercise of power-over does not have to be negative. State legislation to control the spread of diseases, to impose fines for unhealthy behaviour such as smoking in a public place, or even to redistribute market income to prevent poverty, are all examples of what we consider 'healthy' power-over.

Power-over can take different forms and has three functionally distinct operations:

1 dominance, or the direct power to control people's choices, usually by force or its threat;
2 exploitation, or the indirect power to control people's choices through economic relations, in which those who control capital also have control over those who do not; and
3 hegemony, or the ability of a dominant group to control the actions and behaviours of others by intense persuasion (Wrong, 1988).

Power-with

Power-with describes a relationship in which power-over is deliberately used to increase other people's power-from-within and power-over, rather than to dominate or exploit them (Laverack, 2004). To enable others to empower themselves can begin from the perspective to look for, and work from, areas in people's lives in which they are relatively powerful. For example, the female residents of a rooming house in Toronto, Canada, complained of men demanding sexual favours in exchange for letting them gain access to the bathroom. The women requested assistance from the community nurse, who advised the women that, after her initial assistance, they would have to pursue the issue themselves. In this way the nurse strengthened the power-from-within of the women, first by using her status and authority and then by supporting them to act as their own advocates. But in laying aside her power-over condition she exercised her power with the intent of increasing the power-from-within of the women in the relationship (Labonte, 1998). Rather than a simple transfer of resources and information, power-with involves an offering of advice and strategies to develop both the power-from-within of people and the collective empowerment of communities.

Key texts

Laverack, G. (2004) *Health promotion practice: Power and empowerment*. London: Sage Publications.
Laverack, G. (2009) *Public health: Power, empowerment & professional practice*. 2nd edition. London: Palgrave Macmillan.
Scott, J. (2001) *Power*. Cambridge: Polity Press.

Salutogenesis

Salutogenesis describes an approach focusing on factors that support human health and wellbeing, rather than on factors that cause disease. More specifically, the approach is concerned with the relationships between health, stress and coping (Antonovsky, 1979).

The term salutogenesis was developed by the American medical sociologist Aaron Antonovsky. His theories rejected the traditional medical dichotomy separating health and illness and instead described the relationship as a health-ease versus dis-ease continuum (Antonovsky, 1979). The word salutogenesis derives from the Latin *salus* (health) and the Greek *genesis* (origin). Antonovsky developed the term from his studies of how people manage stress and stay well, and he observed that, whilst stress was ubiquitous, not all individuals had negative health outcomes. Instead, some people achieved health despite their exposure to potentially disabling stress factors. In his theory, whether a stress factor was pathogenic, neutral or salutary depended on what he called 'Generalized Resistance Resources' (GRRs). A GRR is any coping resource that is effective in avoiding or combating a range of psychosocial stressors: resources such as money, ego-strength and social support.

Antonovsky's formulation was that the GRRs enabled individuals to make sense of and manage events in their lives. He argued that over time, in response to positive experiences provided by the successful use of different GRRs, an individual would develop an attitude that was in itself the essential tool for coping with stress (Antonovsky, 1979).

> In comparison with resilience, where the conditions and mechanisms are more rigid and contextual, salutogenesis has its strength in adaptability and a focus on problem-solving.

The 'sense of coherence' (SOC) is a theoretical formulation that provides a central explanation for the role of stress in human functioning. In Antonovsky's formulation, the SOC has three components:

1 *Comprehensibility:* a belief that things happen in an orderly and predictable fashion and a sense that you can understand events in your life and reasonably predict what will happen in the future.
2 *Manageability:* a belief that you have the skills or ability, the support, the help or the resources necessary to take care of things, and that things are manageable and within your control.
3 *Meaningfulness:* a belief that things in life are interesting and a source of satisfaction, that things are really worth it and that there is good reason or purpose to care about what happens.

The third element (meaningfulness) is the most important. If a person believes there is no reason to persist and survive and confront challenges, if they have no sense of meaning, then they will have no motivation to comprehend and manage events. The essential argument is that salutogenesis depends on experiencing a strong sense of coherence and that this can lead to positive health outcomes (Lindström and Eriksson, 2005).

Key texts

Antonovsky, A. (1979) *Health, stress and coping*. San Francisco: Jossey-Bass Publishers.

Lindström, B. and Eriksson, M. (2005) Salutogenesis. *Journal of Epidemiology and Community Health*. 59(6): 440–442.

Lindström, B. and Eriksson, M. (2010) *The hitchhiker's guide to salutogenesis: Salutogenic pathways to health promotion*. Helsinki: Fokhälsan Health Promotion Research.

3 | Five useful methods in health promotion

In Chapter 3 I examine five key methods central to health promotion: asset-based community development, harm reduction, innovative communication technologies, lobbying, and moral suasion. Each entry has been included because it can help field workers to better implement empowerment approaches in health promotion programmes. Further information for each entry is provided as key texts to encourage the reader to gain a more in-depth understanding of the subject.

Asset-based community development

Asset-based community development (ABCD) is a methodology that seeks to use the strengths within communities as a means for more sustainable development (Kretzmann and McKnight, 1996).

Asset-based community development is based on the assumption that even the poorest neighbourhood is a place where individuals and organisations represent resources upon which to rebuild (Kretzmann and McKnight, 1996). ABCD is defined by three main characteristics:

1 Asset-based starts with what is present in the community, not with what is absent, needed or problematic, so it aims to uncover the capacities in the community.
2 Internally focused, it concentrates first of all upon the agenda-building and problem-solving capacities of local residents, local associations and local institutions.
3 Relationship driven, it seeks to constantly build and re-build linkages among local people, local institutions and local organisations.

Building on the skills of residents, the power of local associations, and the supportive functions of local institutions, ABCD aims to draw upon existing strengths. The first step in the process is to identify existing, but often unrecognised, assets, and to assess the resources of a community to determine what types of skills and experience are available. The key is to begin to use what is already in the community. The next step is to discover what people in the community care enough about to act on. The final step is to determine how citizens can act together to achieve their goals.

At the core of ABCD is its focus on social relationships. By treating relationships as assets, ABCD is a practical application of the concept of social capital. Social capital in the form of trust, social norms of reciprocity and cooperation resides in relationships and therefore in social networks. Active participation within social networks builds the trust and cohesiveness between individuals that are important to mobilise and create the resources necessary to support collective action.

Justifying the use of an assets-based approach implies that community development has been deficit-based, focusing on what is wrong in communities such as crime, poverty and poor housing. ABCD is politically convenient because it shifts the focus from the realities of inequality and injustice. However, it doesn't ignore these, but instead runs the risk of being seen as the application of superficial government-funded interventions rather than as addressing the real causes of poverty and powerlessness (Harris, 2011).

Key texts

Foot, J. and Hopkins, T. (2010) *A glass half full: How an asset approach can improve community health and well-being.* London: Improvement and Development Agency (IDeA).

Harris, K. (2011) Isn't all community development assets based? *The Guardian online.* Posted 23 June 2011.

Kretzmann, J. P. and McKnight, J. L. (2007) Asset-based community development. *National Civic Review.* 85(4): 23–29.

Harm reduction

Harm reduction is an approach to reduce the harmful consequences of high-risk behaviours by incorporating strategies that cover safer use, managed use and abstinence (Ritter and Cameron, 2006).

People who live in high-risk conditions, and who internalise this as psychosocial risk factors, are more likely to have unhealthier lifestyles, or associated behavioural risk factors – for example, smoking and alcohol consumption. These high-risk behavioural factors can serve as stress-coping rewards even though they can increase susceptibility to a specific cause of illhealth. Even if people living in poor conditions do manage to change their unhealthy behaviours, without any change in their risk conditions, their self-reported health can actually worsen (Blaxter, 2010).

Health and risk behaviours are often related in clusters in a more complex pattern referred to as 'lifestyles'. People caught in this cycle of risk conditions and risk factors can also experience less social support and are less likely to be active in social networks concerned with improving risk conditions in the first place. This further reinforces their sense of isolation and self-blame, confounding the experience of disease or a lack of wellbeing.

Harm-reduction programmes can be contentious because they include issues such as needle exchange, opioid substitution therapy and nicotine substitution. Some government agencies feel that funding should be diverted away from groups that engage in these types of harmful and high-risk behaviours. However, the principles of harm reduction are firmly rooted in humanistic ideals, in the need for immediate goals and the recognition that risky behaviours have always been and always will be a part of society (Ritter and Cameron, 2006).

> The primary goal of harm reduction is to work with people on their terms, in their context and not to condemn their harmful behaviours.

In contrast to harm reduction, the moral approach to addiction tends to enhance the user's shame, guilt and feelings of stigma. The harm-reduction approach is based on acceptance and the willingness of the health promoter to collaborate with others in the course of reducing any harmful consequences (Marlatt and Witkiewitz, 2010).

Harm minimisation is often used interchangeably with harm reduction. However, any intervention or policy that is intended to reduce harmful behaviour can be considered harm reducing. The term harm minimisation is intended to reflect an overall goal of policies to minimise harm (Weatherburn, 2009).

One harm reduction intervention used brief motivational interviews to reduce alcohol-related consequences among adolescents (aged 18–19 years) treated in an emergency room following an alcohol-related event. An assessment of their condition, the future risk of harm and motivational interviews were conducted in the emergency room during or after the patient's treatment. Follow-up assessments showed that patients who received the motivational interviews had a significantly lower incidence of drinking and driving, traffic violations, alcohol-related injuries, and alcohol-related problems than patients who only received the standard care at the emergency room (Monti et al., 1999).

There is widespread evidence that harm-reduction programmes can be effective and cost-efficient, for example, in slowing down the spread of HIV, overdose prevention programmes, emergency room screening and workplace substance use prevention (Marlatt and Witkiewitz, 2010). However, harm reduction is most viable as an approach when it is used in combination with other strategies, such as peer education, to manage high-risk behaviours.

Key Texts

Marlatt, G. A. and Witkiewitz, K. (2010) Update on harm-reduction policy and intervention research. *Annual Review of Clinical Psychology.* 6: 591–606.

Marlatt, G. A., Larimer, M. E. and Witkiewitz, K. (2011) *Harm reduction: Pragmatic strategies for managing high-risk behaviors.* 2nd edition. New York: Guilford Press.

Weatherburn D. (2009) Dilemmas in harm minimization. *Addiction.* 104(3): 335–339.

Innovative communication technologies

In a rapidly changing media environment, health promoters have to continue to take advantage of new technology to better communicate, to organise, to mobilise, to lever for more influence and to raise resources. Innovative communication technologies can be used to reach people at a broad level in civil society and include the Short Message Service and the World Wide Web. The tactics available to health promoters allow the sharing of contacts for better networking and the rapid dissemination of information. The maintenance of a website is also an important tool for information-sharing, organising and mobilisation, and to provide a public profile for health movements and pressure groups (Biddix and Han Woo, 2008).

Innovative communication technology has removed the physical barriers to communication; for example, people are able to participate online in discussions that are classified by topic, each with many conversational threads from across the globe. Online communities, like traditional forms of community, consist of a diverse group of people, but in this case they participate in virtual spaces with little social context and member identity. Social media can encourage communication by enabling participants to find others with whom they share interests and by providing a means to contact them. This facilitates social interactions in online communities and promotes communication by creating chat spaces similar to those that would be created in a room in the offline world. The Internet has helped to promote 'global communities' and 'digital cities' by building arenas in which people can interact and share knowledge and mutual interests. However, online activity is still limited to those who are computer literate and have access to a computer, to the Internet and to a reliable source of electricity, and this can exclude many people (Nomura and Ishida, 2003).

The Short Message Service

The Short Message Service (SMS) allows the interchange of text messages between mobile telephones and is the most widely used data application internationally. The capacity of the mobile telephone to organise people, or to record and publish images of, for example, protests, has already been established. Mobile telephones can also extend participation, monitoring and transparency, decentralise networks and provide opportunities for local innovation. The essential element is not high technology, but universality. Kubatana is a social and political action initiative in Zimbabwe that began on the Internet, but to extend its reach adapted 'FrontlineSMS' to send out regular news updates to people who had either no news source at all, or none that was trustworthy. It was soon discovered that the system was valued for its capacity to operate as a genuine information exchange, putting people from across the country in touch with one another (Banks et al., 2010).

The World Wide Web

The World Wide Web is an important source of specific health information; for example, a survey of over 500 users who went online for healthcare information found that 93 per cent were looking for a specific illness or condition and 65 per cent were looking for information about nutrition, exercise or weight control (Fox and Rainie, 2001). Another survey of 1,700 patients in the UK accessing a health information website showed a high patient demand for online health services such as booking GP appointments and ordering repeat medication. Almost half of the respondents (47%) were aged over 55, indicating that demand for Internet-based health services is not limited to younger patients, and over three-quarters of respondents (78%) were female (Patient UK, 2012).

Health promoters have taken advantage of the World Wide Web and the Internet to become better communicators and social networkers using, for example, Facebook to better inform people. These media communication tools have helped to extend participation, monitoring and transparency, to decentralise networks and to provide opportunities to target individuals about specific health issues.

Key texts

Glaser, J. and Salzberg, C. (2011) *The strategic application of information technology in health care organisations.* San Francisco: Jossey Bass.

Noar, S. M. and Grant-Harrington, N. (2012) *eHealth applications: Promising strategies for behaviour change.* New York: Routledge.

Rohlinger, D. A. and Brown, J. (2009) Democracy, action and the internet after 9/11. *American Behavioural Scientist.* 53(1): 133–150.

Lobbying

Lobbying is the attempt to influence official decisions through the direct and personal communication between a lobbyist and the policymaker (McGrath, 2007).

Lobbying has been criticised on the grounds that it affords undue influence over public policy to powerful and resourced interests at the expense of those groups that are less favoured. Others see lobbying as the manifestation of freedom of expression and a mechanism by which people are able to communicate directly with elected representatives. In practice, lobbying is a feature of the policy-making process in every democratic system and lobbyists commonly describe themselves as forming a bridge between government and the governed. Information from lobbyists can help policy decisions to be better informed and allows people to interact with policymakers more frequently. This can be an important input at the beginning of the policy-making process (see chapter 9). If a policymaker hears from a range of lobbyists on an issue, they will be better informed about the issue and thus better able to reach a position on it. This should not imply, however, that lobbying is a wholly unrestricted activity. Most lobbying is directed at those policymakers who already favour a group's interests or at those who have not yet arrived at a firm view on an issue, rather than being aimed at persuading a policymaker to radically change his or her mind (McGrath, 2007).

Grassroots lobbying is based on the idea that all politics is local, that the more constituents who write or call about an issue, the more likely their elected representatives are to pay attention to it. Crucial to the effectiveness of a grassroots lobbying effort is not the number of constituent communications generated, however, but that all communications demonstrate the same individual voter's genuine views. Grassroots lobbying uses tactics such as e-petitions to raise their concerns to elected officials to express a view about a given forthcoming policy decision.

Not in my backyard (NIMBY) and Nimbyism are used to describe the opposition by people, often local residents, to a proposal for a new development such as a landfill site or airport in their neighbourhood (Hull, 1988).

Counter-tactics by commercial and corporate interests

Many large commercial and corporate health lobbies have far more influence than ordinary citizens, pressure groups or health promotion agencies. Corporations use a range of public relations tactics designed to influence decision-makers, researchers, public opinion and policy analysis (Hager, 2009). There are sophisticated public relations companies specialising in these types of counter-tactics in support of, and often only within the financial reach of, large corporations.

Corporate media campaigns employ sophisticated media management companies to help define and shape issues using well-funded advertising campaigns. A major part of this type of public relations work is attacking opponents and trying to stop them having a 'voice', such as persistently targeting public health researchers working on a specific issue in a way that intimidates them and distracts them from their work. Meanwhile, these companies cultivate and support favourable researchers by providing helpful funding, along with opportunities to travel and to attend conferences. Corporations also routinely seek community or professional groups as 'third parties' to give credibility to their messages publicly. False scientific and community groups have also become an alternative 'tool' that quickly emerge to support large developments or to defend unpopular corporations such as smokers' rights groups. Frequently the lobby groups present themselves publicly as independent and/or science-based; for example, pharmaceutical companies will establish consumer and patient groups in pursuit of their own interests or engage with existing groups in the debate on policy proposals to add legitimacy to their activities (Allsop et al., 2004). The well-resourced interest groups can hire lawyers to put pressure on planned or existing government policies by threatening time-consuming legal action. Another 'tool' of influence is election donations. In New Zealand, for example, the alcohol and tobacco industry has been funding political parties and gaining influence since the early twentieth century (Hager, 2009). There are also corporate gifts where politicians and other targeted people of influence are given, for example, free tickets to big sports games, concerts and cultural events provided by industry interests. Some industries are more aggressive than others; generally the more controversial they are, the more they have to hide or the more negative externalities of their business, the more resources go into these tactics. Some corporations use sponsorship for low-cost marketing such as paying trivial sums for school road-crossing jackets with logos displayed on them, advertising, community events or providing grants for community development activities.

Corporate social responsibility (CSR) – also called corporate conscience, corporate citizenship, social performance, or responsible business – is a form of self-regulation integrated into a business plan or model. CSR policy functions as a built-in mechanism whereby a business monitors and ensures its active compliance with the spirit of the law, ethical standards and international best practices. The goal of CSR is to embrace responsibility for the company's actions and encourage a positive impact through its activities. Promoting CSR reports has become one of the growth areas in the corporate public relations industry. Companies have formed specialist CSR practice groups with the role of embracing accountability and transparency as a means to build corporate credibility and reputation. For example, manufacturing companies that have been criticised for employing child labour, thus potentially damaging their 'corporate image', have devoted much greater attention to developing, overseeing and reporting on new labour standards of suppliers and their sub-contractors as part of a counter-campaign (Knudsen, 2007).

Key texts

Levine, B. (2008) *The art of lobbying: Building trust and selling policy.* Washington, DC: CQ Press.

Libby, P. (2011) *The lobbying strategy handbook: 10 steps to advancing any cause effectively.* London: Sage.

McGrath, C. (2007) Lobbying. In G. L. Andersen and K. G. Herr (eds) 2007 *Encyclopedia of activism and social justice.* London: Sage.

Moral suasion

Moral suasion is the act of trying to use moral principles to influence individuals and groups to change their practices, beliefs and actions (Laverack, 2013b).

Moral suasion is a form of persuasion based on moral reasoning to change people's beliefs and behaviours. Persuasion is a process aimed at changing individual or group attitudes, beliefs or behaviours towards some other event or idea by using methods of communication to convey information, feelings or reasoning, or by using one's personal or positional resources to gain leverage to change other people's behaviours or attitudes (Seiter and Gass, 2010).

The temperance movement

The temperance movement used a strategy of moral suasion to oppose the drinking of alcohol to the point of total abstinence in the UK in the 19th century. The strategy concentrated on the establishment of a mass movement of mostly working men to take a 'pledge' to cease from the use of alcohol. The movement offered support through self-help groups and worked across the classes in society advocating for a sober workforce as well as for 'teetotallers' everywhere (Berridge, 2007).

Foot-binding in China

Foot-binding was universally practised in China; it was painful and dangerous, and it afflicted Chinese women for a millennium. And yet this practice ended, for the most part, within a single generation. The natural-foot movement was championed by liberal modernisers and women's rights advocates and developed in the years of change culminating in the 'Revolution of 1911'. Reform and urban economic development were part of modernisation and mass migration from the countryside. This consequently provided alternative opportunities of support for women, strengthening their independence and bargaining power. The natural-foot movement used moral suasion by forming alliances, called 'pledge associations', of parents who promised not to foot-bind their daughters nor let their sons marry foot-bound women (Mackie, 1996) as moral principles for the basis of individual behaviour change.

Female genital mutilation

An important element in the process of mobilising communities in the fight against female genital mutilation (FGM) is moral suasion and public declarations of the collective decision to abandon the practice. Public declarations can take different forms, including signing a statement, alternative rites-of-passage celebrations, and multi-village gatherings. When public declarations are made, this suggests that a sufficient number of individuals have decided, on moral grounds, not to have their children cut and to abandon FGM, which can further promote broad-scale abandonment. The public declarations, then, can mark a final decision to abandon FGM or are a milestone that signifies readiness for change, and indicates that further support is needed to sustain and accelerate the process (Johansen et al., 2013). Tostan (break through) is a Senegal-based non-governmental organisation (NGO) working for positive social transformation and the abolition of FGM that has had some success in Africa at the community, national and international levels. Tostan has made claims that among women with uncut girls, the rate of women reporting they did not have the intention to cut their daughter was three times higher in areas where Tostan is active than in control villages. The success has been attributed to a strategy supported by strong leadership and a recognition that through, for example, moral suasion and public declarations, people can empower themselves (Gillespie and Melching, 2010).

Moral suasion is a low-cost method that can be used by health promotion practitioners when working with individuals and groups. The limitation of this method is that it focuses on targeting individual behaviour change rather than broader structural change. However, moral suasion can lead on to collective action for the leverage of more favourable government policy.

Key texts

Berridge, V. (2007) Public health activism. *British Medical Journal.* 335: 1310–1312.

Johansen, E., Diop, N., Laverack, G. and Leye, E. (2013) What works and what does not: A discussion of popular approaches for the abandonment of Female Genital Mutilation. *Obstetrics and Gynaecology International.* Advance access ID 348248.

Mackie, G. (1996) Ending foot-binding and infibulation: A convention account. *American Sociological Review.* 61(6): 999–1017.

PART II
Health promotion programmes

4 | Programme management

Health promotion can be delivered as a programme, a project, an intervention or as specific activities. I have used the term 'programme' to cover the different types of delivery and the different stages of delivery. The different stages have to be properly managed, usually by one or more managers, who act as the interface between different partners, administrators and human resource personnel, and who are responsible for budgeting, training, equipment procurement and reporting. Programme management in health promotion requires a multi-disciplinary workforce and is usually performed by 'experts' that are felt to have the necessary professional competencies. This is to ensure that the programme is delivered on time, on budget and in accordance with its aims and objectives.

Programme management in health promotion

The programme management of health promotion has an increasing emphasis on evidence-based practice. Consequently, there has been a reluctance to transfer responsibility to other partners who are perceived as having a different set of competencies, even though, for example, community members are still expected to cooperate with and contribute towards the programme. Managers can underestimate the existing strengths, assets, knowledge and capacities of local partners. This can be further confounded when the managers are involved in cross-cultural programmes and do not consider the resilience of cultural values, the resistance of host institutions, and resentment and mistrust among local partners (Leach, 1994).

> At the heart of a successful health promotion programme is who controls the way in which it is designed, implemented, managed and evaluated.

An empowering approach consciously involves the local partners by including them in its activities and by fostering a sense of ownership. The role of the management is to systematically build the capacity, knowledge and skills of the local partners. One of the first steps towards achieving this is to have clearly defined roles and responsibilities for those involved in the programme. During the planning stage the needs of local partners should be assessed and included in the aims of the programme. Health promotion planning and needs assessment are discussed in detail in chapter 5.

Language and a reflexive practice

Awareness of the use of professional language and of being sensitive to the position and perceptions of others is termed a 'reflexive practice' in which managers are critical about the way they work. When working with other partners, managers often have an advantage through the language that they choose to use as this can either strengthen or weaken the working relationship. Technical terms are a part of the everyday language of managers and have evolved as knowledge and skills develop within a professional subculture. However, the use of specialist language is often confusing both to laypeople and to practitioners not part of the professional subculture. This can contribute to their sense of powerlessness by showing a lack of access to knowledge and the 'expert' power of the person using the technical language.

> Whilst it may sometimes be necessary to use specific technical terms it is better to use a professional language that is understood by everyone.

Scrambler (1987) provides the example of a consultation between a health practitioner and a pregnant woman. The practitioner began the discussion using 'lay' terms to describe the complications associated with her condition, but quickly switched to a technical language when her advice was challenged by the pregnant woman. The woman was then coerced into complying with the practitioner because she suddenly felt uncertain and lacking in knowledge. The pregnant woman had been disempowered by the practitioner, who said that she was unaware of her switch to a more technical language.

The programme cycle

Health promotion programmes can involve a variety of different stages or phases, often dependent on the requirements of the funding agency. However, the programme cycle typically involves four key stages (see figure 4.1):

1 Programme planning, including needs assessment and objective setting (chapter 5);

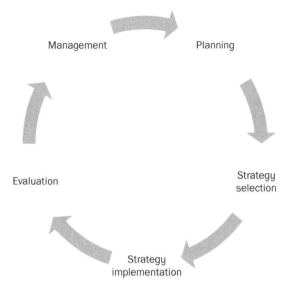

Figure 4.1 The programme cycle

2 Strategy selection, including an identification of programme partners (chapter 6);
3 Strategy implementation with individuals and groups (chapter 7) and communities (chapter 8); and
4 Evaluation (chapter 10).

The different stages also have to be properly managed, with the regular reporting of activities including an analysis of what is working and what is not working. Regular reporting is a standard procedure but varies according to the time period that is covered, including monthly, quarterly, six-monthly, annual, mid-term and end-of-programme feedback. It may seem like a bureaucratic task, but regular reporting serves an important function, including accountability to funders, maintaining the trust and support of partners and allowing changes to be made to the programme to make it more effective and efficient. Each programme will have its own reporting procedure and style, and whilst the information may come from several different sources, such as from various technical staff, it will usually be the responsibility of the manager to collate, analyse and write the final report.

Budget considerations

The programme budget provides an estimate of how much money is planned to be spent to achieve its aims and objectives. The budget is usually itemised using 'budget headings' in regard to specific programme costs such as administration, training, technical services, materials, equipment and transport. The planned expenditures are provided over specific periods such as monthly, quarterly, six-monthly or annual costs and cover the total programme duration.

> In practice there is often little flexibility in the budget, and once it has been approved it is unlikely to be modified or extended to meet changing expectations.

Once the budget has been agreed during the design stage of the programme it is often difficult to change, and any new activities that are not covered can be rejected. To overcome this, some programmes have a more flexible budget design: for example, to have a percentage of funds under an 'open' heading to allow other activities to be implemented. This is sometimes called a 'slush fund'. Alternatively, the programme management can be given permission to use a proportion of the budget (to an agreed amount) for unforeseeable circumstances or activities that arise as the programme develops.

Managers as enablers

The qualities of an enabling relationship in programme management would include a non-coercive dialogue in the identification of needs, using professional status to give credibility and to strengthen the role of the local partners. The range of skills that programme managers require include team building, using democratic decision-making processes, and conflict resolution. Programme managers often play an important role by providing infrastructural support, skills development, raising the level of critical awareness of other partners, and the provision of finances. Their role is essentially to enable the partners of the programme to gain more ownership and control by discovering their own capabilities. Programme management and leadership skills are therefore closely linked; however, good leaders do not necessarily have good organisational skills and may lack management experience.

Leadership skills in programme management

The qualities of good leadership in programme management include being charismatic, visionary, passionate and reflexive. Typologies of competency, the ways in which a good leader puts his or her skills into practice, place an emphasis on motivating, inspiring, collaborating,

communicating and empowering. Good leaders are aware of the efforts
of others, use a reflexive practice to be creative and are able to adapt
to challenges (Frusciante, 2007). Good leadership involves both personal and organisational qualities and characteristics such as a decision-
making style, networking and political efficacy. Effective leaders also
manage time properly and maintain ongoing involvement of all the members of the programme.

> Leadership can be described as a process of social influence in which
> one person can enlist the aid and support of others in the accomplish-
> ment of a shared task. A leader is often seen as somebody whom peo-
> ple follow, who guides or directs others (Chemers, 1997).

Mechanisms must exist to ensure the continuity of vision even after a
leader has left, to avoid losing the impetus of the programme. One solution is to select a mix of different types of leaders or else make a conscious
commitment to sharing power: for example, consensus decision-making,
and encouraging everyone to play a variety of roles in the programme.
Leadership still exists in such groups, but it is leadership based on contributions and respect, not formal roles (Martin, 2007). However, a proper
balance between leadership and lay decision-making is essential because
conflict can occur when there is a lack of clarity regarding who has
authority (Anderson et al., 2006).

> Simply put, an effective leader must also be a good manager and
> organiser, and is the person who decides what needs to be done and
> then gets people to do it.

In the absence of good leadership a steering group, task force or committee can be a useful way to maintain the strategic direction of the
programme. This provides regular feedback and is an opportunity to
reflect and act on the lessons learnt and to follow up on recommendations (Smithies and Webster, 1998).

Professional competencies

Health promotion practitioners are expected to display a specialisation
of knowledge, technical competence, social responsibility and service.
Their level of professionalism is attained through education, training,

professional codes of practice and core competencies. Core competencies provide a set of standards by which the workforce can determine what a 'professional' practice is, and can be used to set parameters for staff development, recruitment and performance (Laverack, 2007). However, for some practitioners the activity of health promotion is only a part of their daily work: for example, a nurse who undertakes a mix of clinical practice and health education. Different professional groups have therefore developed their own sets of competencies to provide a minimum entry level to meet a professional standard. For practitioners who are not solely involved in health promotion it is the responsibility of their profession to select which specialist competencies they feel are most relevant to their work.

> Competencies are a combination of knowledge, skills and values that enable an individual to perform a set of tasks to an appropriate standard (Dempsey et al., 2011).

An international meeting to identify core competencies, core values and principles for health promotion identified eight domains that are required to engage in effective practice:

1 Catalysing change;
2 Leadership;
3 Assessment;
4 Planning;
5 Implementation;
6 Evaluation;
7 Advocacy; and
8 Partnerships (Barry et al., 2009).

Another set of six core competencies is given in table 4.1 and although not exhaustive it does provide examples of what is required to allow health promotion practitioners to grow and develop their professional standards (Laverack, 2007).

Conflict resolution

> Conflict resolution is involved in facilitating the peaceful ending of conflict by actively communicating information about differing motives or ideologies and by engaging in collective negotiation (Forsyth, 2009).

Table 4.1 Core competencies for health promoters

Core competency	Description
Programme design, management, implementation and evaluation	The ability to plan effective health promotion programmes, including the management of resources and personnel. This involves an understanding of programme cycles, budgeting, and the planning and evaluation of bottom-up approaches in top-down programming.
The planning and delivery of effective communication strategies	Communication strategies are an integral part of many health promotion programmes to increase knowledge levels and to raise awareness. A high level of competence is needed for the development of programmes that target individuals, groups and communities, including one-to-one communication, the design of print materials and the use of the mass media.
Facilitating skills	Good facilitation skills – for example, for training or running meetings and advisory groups – are essential for health promoters and are an important part of programme design.
Research skills	Health promotion programme design and evaluation is based on sound research including the use of participatory techniques, qualitative and quantitative methods, and systematic reviews.
Community capacity-building skills	Community empowerment is central to health promotion. This is a process of capacity-building, and health promoters must be competent in a range of strategies that they can use to help individuals, groups and communities to gain more power.
Ability to influence policy and practice	Health promoters have the opportunity to influence policy and practice in their everyday work: for example, through technical advisory groups and through helping communities to mobilise and organise themselves towards gaining power.

Conflict can be a negative ingredient of health promotion programmes by taking attention away from important issues, by dividing groups and by undermining individual positions. However, if managed correctly it can also be a positive ingredient. Dealing with conflict in a positive way can resolve disputes, help to release emotions and anxieties, and help people to address sensitive issues whilst at the same time improving cooperation. The beginnings of conflict are often caused by poor communication between individual partners, weak leadership, internal struggles to gain access to limited resources and the uncertainty of roles and responsibility (Laverack, 2009). The programme manager can play an important role in resolving conflict by simply assessing the situation, being a good listener and inviting partner participation to clarify areas of conflict.

The Aik Saath project

The Aik Saath project was started to address inter-ethnic tension and outbreaks of conflict between Sikh and Muslim youth in Slough, UK. The role of locally recruited and trained facilitators in conflict resolution played a major role in reducing tensions, such as the number of playground fights between Sikhs and Muslims, and in building a working relationship with street gangs. The project also used local conflict resolution groups and worked in schools to identify and address the key issues causing the tensions. The conflict resolution groups were made up of students from each year and provided an important entry point into the school and into the issues facing youth around inter-ethnic conflict. The groups provided a bridge between the practitioners and the youth and so it was important to carefully manage their development. The project found that in order to develop a conflict resolution group it was necessary to carefully select the targeted youth, to work with existing community-based organisations in contact with the youth and to invest in young people to act as facilitators. These people were then provided with outreach resources and helped to engage with key public sector agencies to achieve their aims (renewal.net, 2008).

Conflict resolution does not have to be a specialist area of work, especially when the issue of disagreement is uncomplicated and may be resolved through a clarification and discussion of the main concerns. Conflict resolution can be facilitated by using participatory approaches (see below) to firstly, define and map the main issues held between the different partners involved, and then by developing strategies to discuss and address each concern.

Defining the issues of conflict

To carry out this technique for conflict resolution, the facilitator should have information about the key questions that will be asked and some of the solutions that can be discussed. This will help to focus the discussion on the practical and not on the personal and in neutral terms that all participants can agree upon, as follows:

1 The participants are asked to construct a list of key questions about the conflict, and the potential solutions to the questions.
2 The participants and the facilitator next identify sources of information regarding each of the key questions – for example, websites, local leaders, government officials – that are necessary to move into a problem-solving stage.
3 The participants are asked to prepare a summary of the conflict by comparing each question with a possible solution, which can be usefully summarised in a table.
4 After a period of discussion between the different parties the summary can be rewritten to highlight how major changes in one conflict can change over time as circumstances change.

This type of a problem-solving technique is simply an agreement towards further analysis and discussion. There are a number of other different approaches for conflict resolution that are more complex: notably, negotiation, mediation, diplomacy and creative peace-making (Mitchell and Banks, 1998).

Using an ethical approach in programme management

Ethics is the branch of philosophy dealing with distinctions between right and wrong and with the moral consequences of human actions (PHAC, 2013).

Central to an ethical approach to health promotion is the concept of empowerment. Per-Anders Tengland (2007), a prominent health promotion philosopher, believes that the logic for using an empowering approach is justified because it is well founded, and ethically and morally sound to do so. Tengland concludes from a conceptual analysis that empowerment has applicability for creating freedom and opportunity to improve health. However, he questions if most practitioners have the knowledge and skills that are required to undertake an ethical approach to their work. Managers, for example, often work with people from different cultural backgrounds and need to have a shared understanding of the issues if they are to use empowering approaches in their everyday work. This would include a better understanding of themselves, their beliefs and values, and putting this into a framework of the relevant social and cultural perceptions, to respect and to focus on central conditions in people's lives that support autonomy (Seedhouse, 1997).

> Programme managers have a responsibility to use an ethical approach to their work and to promote autonomy: doing good and not harming others.

A key ethical tension in health promotion is whether people actually do want to gain more control over their lives, health and its determinants. In practice, it is the manager, or their agency, that usually initiates the programme and provides the initial enthusiasm for its direction. This is contradictory to an empowering approach in which the issue to be addressed and the means of reaching a solution should be led by the partners of the programme, based on their needs.

Key ethical issues raised in regard to programme management include strong paternalism, coercion and manipulation, and, in particular, not respecting personal autonomy. Autonomy refers to the capacity to be self-governing, to make the decisions that will influence one's life and health. It is linked to what it is to be a person, to be able to choose freely and to be able to formulate how one wants to live one's life. It is also related to having the freedom and opportunities in our lives to be able to make the right choices for ourselves (Laverack, 2013a: 58).

Another ethical issue in programme management refers to 'blaming' others by placing an emphasis on individual responsibility when it is wrong to think that people are always able to choose healthier lives. People may be powerless to control factors that determine their behaviour (Holland, 2007) such as unemployment. However, those defined as the 'victims' of the blame may identify themselves with this term and feel that they do not have the right or do not possess the motivation to change their circumstances. For those people who refuse or who cannot take responsibility to change their circumstances the programme can play an important role to motivate, to organise and to mobilise others.

Programme sustainability

> Sustainability is the extent to which a programme is able to be continued beyond its implementation period (Macdowall et al., 2006).

Sustainable programmes aim to build healthy public policy and supportive environments for health in ways which improve living conditions, support healthy lifestyles and achieve greater equity in health. Community involvement in the programme is an important aspect of sustainability and includes the partners in decision-making and taking on a sense of ownership. Evidence shows that community involvement has been able to lead to sustained changes linked to improvements in health. For example, in Piha, New Zealand, local action brought about bans on public drinking, resulting in fewer injuries and incidents of crime and an improved sense of wellbeing (Conway, 2002). Elsewhere, community action projects on alcohol regulation have resulted in bar staff training, shortening of the hours of operation of licensed premises, increased age-verification checks and highly visible drink-driving enforcement resulting in reductions in injury (Holder et al., 1997) and in drink-driving in those aged 18–19 years (Wagenaar et al., 2000).

Key factors for programme sustainability

The programme management has an important role to ensure that key factors for sustainability are systematically implemented, including engaging with communities to share their needs, capacity-building, providing flexible funding and being creative to expand on successful initiatives.

Engage communities to share priorities

A major step towards sustainability is to accommodate local agendas within the design of the programme by engaging with communities during the planning phase. Engaging with people is crucial but it is not straightforward; for example, research in the UK has shown that of 80 per cent of people who claimed to want to get involved in a community-based activity only 25 per cent were actually prepared to give up their time to do so (Confederation of British Industry, 2006). Programmes can only be sustainable if they can maintain a high level of participation and motivation among the beneficiaries. Engaging with people to address local needs can be facilitated by using innovative methods (see chapter 5) and is especially important when working with marginalised groups that can become isolated from the programme activities.

Build community capacity

Sustainable programming must have a clearly defined strategy for how it will build community capacity through systematically strengthening knowledge, skills and competencies. Without this focus the partners can become dependent on the programme to provide support and resources without themselves taking responsibility for greater control. The process of building capacity can begin around small-scale initiatives with a view to expand on successful community outcomes. Joan Wharf

Higgins and colleagues (2007) in British Columbia, Canada looked at 11 regional seed-funded initiatives (receiving short-term grants up to 4,500 Canadian dollars) for chronic disease prevention. They found that those initiatives with most capacity-building had a better chance of success, especially if resources could be found for the longer term. The conclusion was that 10 out of the 11 initiatives continued beyond the funded period and that these types of partnerships between communities and government agencies can work towards achieving sustainability.

Mechanisms for flexible funding

The programme should be flexible in the type and timing of resources that it can provide rather than being designated to a specific budget category. These activities may be difficult to justify but nonetheless they build the social dimension of communities through a sense of belonging, connectedness and personal relationships. Funders must therefore be able to think 'outside the box' to provide flexible financial support, for example, for matching counterpart contributions, covering recurrent community costs and providing sufficient contingency funds for unplanned activities.

However, funders are often reluctant to take risks with resources for activities that they feel are unpredictable or which cannot be easily measured. One example that has demonstrated how to reduce resource risks is for the community to establish a joint venture, for example between government, private and public interests, such as the Safer Parks Scheme in Christchurch, New Zealand. The Safer Parks Scheme was started by the City Council following many complaints about crime in public parks. These open areas provided facilities for people to do more exercise such as walking and cycling, and they were not being used because of the fear of attack. The Safer Parks Scheme invested in employing more park wardens and honorary rangers to patrol the areas, installing cycle ways and play equipment for children to make access easier. The Scheme encouraged public participation through its 'adopt a park' initiative and recruited volunteers to help to raise sponsorship money, to provide preservation and protection work and to report any problems that they encountered in the parks. The volunteers and the public attended regular meetings to identify problems, solutions and actions, and as a result of all these activities park patronage increased (Gee, 2008).

Be creative to expand on successful initiatives

Sustainable programmes have to be more creative to scale up or expand upon successful initiatives that address local concerns. Scaling-up across populations has been achieved, for example, in Bangladesh through partnerships such as the Bangladesh Rural Advancement Committee and the Grameen Bank (Papa et al., 2006). Scaling-up remains an important but unresolved issue for many programmes. There is no real agreement on the amount of increase that a programme has to obtain in order to reach a 'scale-up'. However, this is usually considered to be the coverage of benefits to as many of the population within a specified area as possible, more quickly, more equitably and more lastingly. The problem begins when pilot programmes are not planned to be scaled up: for example, by adding a creative initiative to an existing larger programme, even when successful.

Expanding on successful initiatives is important to gain greater benefits but must be sensitive to how to continue to meet local needs at a broader level.

Whether working with existing groups or new ones, in a partnership or directly engaging with the community, the roles and responsibilities of who facilitates the 'scaling-up' process must be clearly defined. Small-scale programmes are often successful because they are structured in such a way as to accommodate complex local needs. 'Going to scale' can result in these dynamics becoming disrupted and roles at a local level not being acknowledged in a meaningful way. The impact, intentional or not, can have an effect on the 'scaling-up' process, for example, through a lack of participation or lower community contributions (Earle et al., 2004).

Key points of the chapter

- It is more empowering to use language that is understood by everyone.
- It is more empowering to use a 'reflexive practice' in which managers are critical about the way they use their influence over others
- An effective leader must also be a good manager and organiser, and is the person who decides what needs to be done and then gets people to do it.
- Programme managers have a responsibility to use an ethical approach to their work and to promote autonomy: doing good and not harming others.
- Funders must be able to think outside the box to provide flexible financial support.
- Sustaining successful initiatives is important to gain greater benefits but must be sensitive to how to continue to meet local needs at a broader level.

5 | Health promotion planning

Programme planning can be made more effective by using strategic and participatory approaches that allow the involvement of the different partners. Rather than being time-limited or one-off the programme then becomes a means through which longer-term capacities can be built. The various financial, material and human resources that are available are used to strengthen the knowledge, skills and competencies of all the programme partners.

Programme design considerations

During the planning process it is important to consider the time frame and size of the programme, as these parameters can often determine if it will be successful or not. It is important, for example, that practitioners appreciate the gradual developmental and sometimes long-term process of a programme, especially one that addresses complex social processes. If the time frame used is too short then these long-term processes run the risk of being ineffective. Similarly, if the programme is too large then the design may not be able to provide sufficient coverage or adequately involve key stakeholders at a local level.

Programme time frame

Health promotion programmes typically have a fixed time frame of 1–3 years, and this is considered to be sufficient to allow its activities, often educational and motivational, to be implemented. There is not a definitive timescale to facilitate the programme partners becoming more empowered, but a longer time frame is necessary to address broader capacity-building and complex social goals, typically 5–7 years. However, an extension of the programme time frame to achieve these goals can be viewed by funding agencies as a failure: as the programme's not having not met its objectives. To overcome this the programme design should have a flexible or extended time frame for some, or all, of its activities.

Some programme outcomes can be achieved within a relatively short time frame; however, as this cannot always be guaranteed an evaluation of the process (as well as the outcome) will provide evidence of continuing successes. Too short a programme time frame runs the real risk of initiating healthy changes, only to end before such changes have reached some degree of sustainability. The result can be an increase in perceived powerlessness by programme partners: for example, a failure to address local needs and a resultant perception of the waste of limited resources (Korsching and Borich, 1997).

A programme should start with realistic objectives that are achievable within a relatively short time frame. The purpose is to produce visible successes, to sustain interest and to promote participation in other more complex initiatives.

Programme size

Health promotion programmes should be designed to initially look critically at local issues that can be best achieved through small-scale initiatives. Later these will need to develop and to grow if they are to effect change in the external environment. The size of a programme should allow aspects of it to be managed by the beneficiaries, many of whom may have little experience and initially few skills. This can be better achieved by focusing on relatively small numbers of people in small programmes, thus avoiding some of the problems associated with large-scale interventions (Laverack, 2004).

Needs assessment

Needs assessment is used to identify the needs reported by an individual, group or community, and the resources and outcomes that are required (Gilmore, 2011).

A needs assessment should be the starting point of every health promotion programme and include an identification of the assets of people and the development of programme activities based on their capabilities, knowledge and skills. Community asset mapping, for example, is an inventory of the strengths of the people and their social interconnections and networks, and of how these can be accessed. This is important because the opportunities for health promotion are to a large extent dependent on social, financial, physical and environmental assets at a local level (Jirojwong and Liamputtong, 2009).

Both the programme and its partners have needs that they may wish to address. Those of the programme are typically based on epidemiological studies and systematic reviews. In contrast, the needs of the partners are typically based on addressing local concerns and problems. Sometimes these two sets of needs are similar and can be reconciled in the design of the programme. More often, the needs are dissimilar and a compromise has to be found through the design and implementation of the programme.

> A needs assessment that includes all partners is a logical starting point in the design of a programme and can build longer-term working relationships.

A needsassessment approach involves quantitative as well as qualitative methods to determine priorities, what should be done, what can be done and what can be afforded. However, too rigid an approach runs the risk of becoming too controlling, whilst too flexible an approach runs the risk of delay or not having a direction with which to move forward (Wright, 2001).

In practice, who will participate in the needs assessment is essentially decided through the representation of a few partners on behalf of the majority: for example, the elected representatives of a community. This is because it is not usually possible for everyone to participate in the needs assessment even when using participatory methods. The diversity of some communities can create problems with regard to the selection of representatives. Participation can become empty and frustrating for those whose involvement is passive. Participation can sometimes allow those in authority – for example, the programme management – to claim that all sides were considered whilst only a few benefit.

Four categories of need

Generally, the process of needs assessment covers four main categories:

1 Normative need is usually set by experts against a standard or norm: for example, welfare benefits.
2 Comparative need is by comparison to others who are not in need: for example, in the selection of the most deprived in society.
3 Felt need is that perceived by people who feel that they have a need.
4 Expressed need is inferred from people's demands: for example, for improved health services (Bradshaw, 1972).

Mapping

Mapping is an important stage in needs assessment and includes engaging with an 'audience': the identification, ranking and prioritisation of their concerns and assets.

Engaging large audiences

There are a number of mapping techniques based on the principles of collaborative needs assessment that can be used to engage a large audience. These include whole-system planning, search conferences, values summits, and Open Space and Big Conversation events. Whilst these approaches may be too large, time consuming and expensive for many practitioners to use it is worthwhile looking at two examples to illustrate how they work in practice: whole-system planning and values summits.

Whole-system planning

Whole-system planning is an approach to bring together many diverse sub-groups and interests to collect information, to understand one another and to build a plan to realign around current and future plans. The event is held in a large space where people can come together, such as in a community centre or events venue. The whole-system planning approach typically follows a process:

1   The first part or day focuses on the past. Attention to the past can be used to also understand the causes of need and if these are still a problem.
2   The next part is focused on the present challenges, strengths and weaknesses.
3   Finally, the third part focuses on the future, often beginning with a visioning exercise to determine a desired future state. This vision is then shared, developed and given local meaning for all involved (Changing minds, 2013).

Values summits

A values summit brings together a diverse range of people and their perspectives to create a better understanding of how people's differences, social status and cultural expectations can affect their experiences of health and health care. They create a space for patients, the public and citizens to connect with leaders and health professionals, and offer a fresh way to talk about, listen to and understand key issues. Values summits typically take two forms: open and closed consultations. Open consultations use informal meetings in, for example, GP waiting rooms, supermarkets and town squares to ask people about their views on a particular health issue. These events are often a partnership approach with the community services provider, voluntary sector and local councils all participating in the organisation. Closed consultations use anonymous online surveys, questionnaires and individual interviews to gain the views of people on a particular health issue (National Health Service, 2013).

Engaging smaller audiences

There are a number of strategies for mapping that can be used within health promotion programmes with small, more manageable groups, and these include asset mapping, citizens' juries and PhotoVoice. The role of the practitioner is to encourage others to think critically about their own assets, their access to external resources and their ability to make decisions (Rifkin and Pridmore, 2001). Once the needs have been identified it is the role of the practitioner to then help others to rank them and to move towards decision-making and action. When practitioners are working with local partners who are non-literate, pictures or drawings can be used instead of words to develop a ranked list. The list can then be scored, placing the highest at the top and the lowest score at the bottom, to help with prioritisation.

Asset mapping

Asset mapping is one of the methods commonly used in asset-based community development (see chapter 3) to mobilise people around a common vision (Kretzmann and McKnight, 1996). Its purpose is to generate an inventory of the resources and capacities available at the individual, group and institutional levels within a given community (Foot and Hopkins, 2010).

Six key community assets

Asset mapping uses six categories (Foot and Hopkins, 2010), based on the assumption that every community has a unique set of skills and capacities:

1 Individual residents of the community have resources, skills and assets that should be recognised and identified.
2 Associations and small informal groups of people, such as clubs and associations, are critical to community mobilisation and an opportunity for people to come together around a common interest based on individual choice.

3 Institutions include paid groups of professionals who are structur-
   ally organised such as government agencies, private business and
   schools. They can be valuable resources and can help the community capture resources and establish a sense of civic responsibility.
4 Physical assets include land, buildings, space and funds that can be
   used by the community.
5 The economic assets of an area include local businesses.
6 The cultural assets of an area include art, culture and expressions of
   creativity.

Community asset mapping

Community asset mapping has received considerable attention in, for
example, the UK, as a way to foster the 'Big Society agenda'. This concerns moving power away from central government and giving it to
local communities and individuals through empowering others, changing and opening up public services and promoting social action (South
et al., 2013).

Guidance (NHS North West, 2011) on how to successfully undertake
a community asset-mapping approach includes:

• The community should identify the assets that they value as these
  are likely to have the greatest impact. Individual and community
  capacities can be considered as assets only in so far as they are valuable to the community.
• It is important to consider what the reasons to do it are and what it is
  hoped will be achieved by it. These considerations are likely to determine the geographic area to be assessed, the size of the sample to be
  interviewed and the questions to be asked in the mapping exercise.
• It is important to consider, early on in the process, how the surveyed
  assets will be hosted such as using a database, as this will affect how
  they may be updated in the future.
• It is important to make sure that the final mapping is continually
  monitored to check whether it is up to date and still useful.
• Asset mapping can be a time-intensive activity that requires good
  planning and resources when undertaken efficiently in a time-
  constrained period. Experience shows that it is important to involve
  a variety of volunteers who can liaise with different segments of
  local communities. Questionnaires can be an efficient way to systematically collect information on people's personal assets; however,
  the questions must be able to reach the correct level of detail, otherwise the answers will have limited usability. Similarly, local events
  can be a successful way to undertake asset mapping and offer a
  context in which to identify specific and individually valued goals
  (Giuntoli et al., 2012).

The Altogether Better project

The Altogether Better project is a collaborative network aimed at building capacity to empower communities to improve their own health and wellbeing. In 2011 the project took a lead in undertaking a community asset-mapping project. The overall aim of the 'I Am My Community' asset mapping was to build capacity in communities and to extend the skills and expertise of local volunteers. The project was undertaken in two disadvantaged communities in Sheffield, Firth Park and Sharrow, in the UK. Four main practical lessons emerged:

1 the importance of securing adequate financial resources to pay for the staff involved in the asset mapping, which proved to be very time intensive;
2 the need to involve a wider pool of volunteers to expand the chances of success of the project;
3 the need to define clear and more specific goals for the asset mapping in order to make it easier to recruit volunteers for its delivery; and
4 the need to collect data on people's personal assets in a systematic way in order for it to be usable (Giuntoli et al., 2012).

Grounded citizens' juries

The grounded citizens' jury is an approach for local involvement in health needs assessment and decision-making. For example, the concerns identified by people in South West Burnley, UK, using this approach included:

• low pay;
• poor housing and an increasing number of empty and derelict properties;
• increasing alcohol abuse by children;
• high crime levels, especially drug-related burglaries;
• poor access to health and social services;
• teenage pregnancies; and
• a high volume of fast-moving traffic and accidents (Kashefi and Mort, 2004).

The process begins when a steering committee selects 12–16 citizens to form the jury. These jury members are selected because they can offer an opinion on the health needs of their community and not because they represent a particular section or organisation. Jury members may be single mothers, the elderly, unemployed or people from an average-sized family, for example. The jury meets for a 4–5 day period with the purpose of reaching a 'verdict' on a particular long-standing problem regarding local circumstances and service provision related to the health needs of its citizens. The jury is posed a general question such as 'what would improve the health and wellbeing of residents in your community?' The jury members undergo a period of training in preparation for the meeting and are given time to asks questions about their roles and responsibilities. The jury hears testimonies from local health and welfare workers, and members are presented with the results of data collected about community opinions such as focus groups with school children. They may meet with local community groups before further deliberation and the preparation of a report. The commissioning agency is committed to respond and take action on some of the recommendations made by the jury. The jury members are not practitioners or researchers and their deliberations can result in many recommendations that cover pertinent local concerns. Prioritisation is therefore an important step in focusing the jury onto a few key needs and the solutions that they are able to recommend, such as improved public transport for the elderly. Follow-up to the jury recommendations and the inclusion of jury members in this process of further development are key points for the success of the approach.

PhotoVoice

PhotoVoice enables people to identify, represent and enhance their community through a specific photographic technique. It entrusts cameras to people to enable them to act as recorders and potential catalysts for social action and change, in their own communities (PhotoVoice, 2013).

PhotoVoice can be used to reach, inform and organise community members, enabling them to prioritise their concerns and discuss problems and solutions. PhotoVoice uses the immediacy of the visual image and accompanying stories to furnish evidence and to promote an effective, participatory means of sharing experiences and local knowledge to resolve problems. It enables people to define for themselves what is worth remembering and what needs to be changed.

PhotoVoice has two main goals:

- to enable people to record and reflect their community's strengths and concerns; and
- to promote critical dialogue and knowledge about personal and community issues through group discussions of photographs (PhotoVoice, 2013).

People using PhotoVoice engage in a three-stage process that provides the foundation for analysing the pictures they have taken:

Stage 1. Selecting: Choosing those photographs that most accurately reflect the community's concerns and assets. So that people can lead the discussion, it is they who choose the photographs. They select photographs they consider most significant, or simply like best, from among those they have taken.

Stage 2. Contextualising or storytelling: The participatory approach also generates the second stage, contextualising or storytelling. This occurs in the process of group discussion, voicing individual and collective experience. People have to describe the meaning of their images in group discussions and it is this that provides meaning and context.

Stage 3. Codifying: The participatory approach gives multiple meanings to single images and thus frames the third stage, codifying. In this stage, participants may identify three types of dimensions that arise from the dialogue process: issues, themes or theories. The individual or group may codify issues when the concerns targeted for action are pragmatic, immediate and tangible.

PhotoVoice can help to engage community members in needs assessment, asset mapping and programme planning.

Having an influence on the broader causes of poverty – for example, unemployment – has not been achieved using PhotoVoice because this requires further action beyond asset mapping including leveraging a political commitment.

Top-down and bottom-up

The way in which health needs are defined and addressed are central to an empowering health promotion approach. Traditionally, health promotion planning can take two distinct forms: bottom-up and top-down.

A bottom-up approach encourages the community to identify its own needs and to communicate these 'upwords' to those with the decision-making authority. Every Australian Counts, for example, used a bottom-up approach in its campaign for a national disability insurance scheme in Australia. The campaign recruited influential people or 'champions' to support its cause, such as media personalities (Every Australian Counts, 2012). This was made easier because people were interested and passionate about the issue of inequality and disability.

The framing of health as individualised can create an obstacle for bottom-up approaches. The personalisation of health provides a focus on the 'struggle', 'fight' or 'battle' against a disease or illness. The emphasis is on self-blame, personal responsibility and individual action. Individuals may be committed to change but this is only at the personal level and does not address the necessity for broader action. People who are passionate, even angry, about climate change, for example, are mobilised to protest about an issue that affects us all. But obesity and heart disease affect us individually, and the response is to deal with these issues at a personal level and not at a community level. The issue is not perceived as a threat to us all and this makes collective action difficult. However, there have been exceptions: for example, the collective action of the gay community in the 1980s to cope with the effects of HIV/AIDS. Such was the determination of this community that the extent of interaction had probably not been seen before in regard to a health issue by both the medical profession and groups within civil society (Brashers et al. 2002). The spread of HIV was perceived as a threat by gay men to other gay men and this motivated many of them to act collectively.

In contrast, top-down describes programmes where needs identification comes from those in authority in top structures 'down' to the community. Top-down programmes would include almost all health education and multi-risk factor reduction interventions such as lifestyle and behaviour approaches. The Multiple Risk Factors Intervention Trial (MRFIT), for example, was a ten-year programme designed to reduce mortality from heart disease in the top 10 per cent male risk group. The trial undertook a large survey of 400,000 men in 22 cities in the USA, and randomly selected 6,000 for the intervention and 6,000 for the control group. The trial was the most ambitious, expensive and intensive anywhere tried at that time. The trial failed and after six years the men in the intervention group did not achieve a lower mortality level from coronary heart disease than men in the control group (Syme, 1997).

Top-down and bottom-up are ideal types of health promotion practice that are used to demonstrate important differences in relation to programme planning that can create a tension. The practitioner 'pushes down' a predefined agenda onto the community that in turn attempts to 'pushup' an agenda based on its needs. This tension can be resolved through parallel-tracking, discussed later in this chapter.

Bottom-up approaches consciously involve the community in the programme and in the planning decisions. In practice, this simply means that the roles and responsibilities of all the programme partners are formally documented and that capacity is systematically built as a part of the design.

A health promotion programme will have a better chance of success if it includes the needs of the people that it is designed to benefit.

Objective setting

In conventional (top-down) health promotion programming, objectives are typically centred on disease prevention and lifestyle management related to a change in specific health behaviours. The objectives are predetermined during the design phase and are based on broader epidemiological studies: for example, population data on the major causes of morbidity and mortality. Local needs (bottom-up) are expressed in a different way – for example, concerns about adolescent drug use – and can change as the programme progresses. The local partners may later decide to narrow its focus towards more immediate and resolvable objectives: for example, to establish youth employment opportunities in a given locality. The challenge in objective setting is to accommodate both top-down and bottom-up objectives in the same health promotion programme. The example of addressing obesity in the Polynesian population in New Zealand helps to illustrate some of the key issues in setting objectives.

Addressing obesity in the Polynesian population

In Auckland, New Zealand, Polynesian people aged 45 years and above have rates for cardiovascular heart disease which are consistently and significantly higher (about twice as high) than those in the total population. Polynesian males and females also have higher prevalence rates for diabetes and worse causal related indicators for obesity, diet, physical exercise and tobacco consumption (Ministry of Health and Pacific Island Affairs, 2004). A top-down health promotion programme to address chronic disease prevention would include objectives to:

- reduce body mass index by X% in X% of the population before end of year XXXX;
- bring blood pressure readings into normal range for X% of the population before end of year XXXX;
- bring cholesterol levels into normal range for X% of the population before end of year XXXX.

Conversely, the identified local needs of local Polynesian communities in Auckland were (Moana, 2005):

- Better facilities for vegetable gardening. A good form of exercise and an activity that people wanted to do, especially the aged.
- Walking groups for women. A means of also building social networks and support groups based around a physical activity.
- More information about diabetes. In both English and Polynesian languages presented through appropriate channels of communication.

The issue at stake is how the top-down track, defined by the agency, and the bottom-up track, identified as community needs, can become linked during the progressive stages of the programme cycle. This requires a fundamental change in the way we think about health promotion programming. 'Parallel-tracking' helps to move our thinking on theoretically from a simple bottom-up/top-down dichotomy and provides a systematic way in which to accommodate the two sets of needs.

Parallel-tracking

Parallel-tracking is a planning framework which uses a multi-stage approach to view the top-down and bottom-up tensions in health

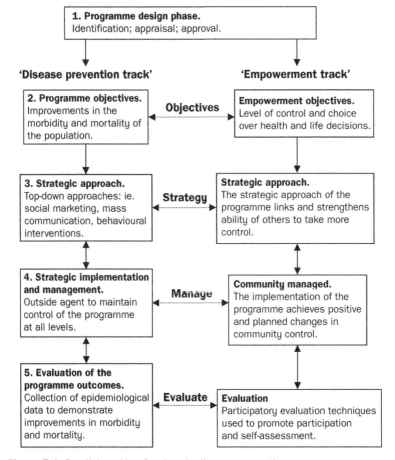

Figure 5.1 Parallel-tracking for chronic disease prevention (Laverack, 2007: 50)

promotion programming in a uniquely different way (Laverack, 2007). Community needs are viewed as a 'parallel track' running alongside the main 'programme track'. The tensions between the two, rather than being conventionally viewed as a top-down versus a bottom-up situation, can now occur at each stage of the programme cycle, making their resolution much easier. The framework can also help to increase community abilities to address the programme activities at each stage of the cycle. Figure 5.1 provides an example of how parallel-tracking can be applied in practice in regard to a health promotion chronic disease programme.

Key points of the chapter

- A health promotion programme has a better chance of success and sustainability if the planning includes the needs of the people that it is designed to benefit.
- Needs assessment that includes all partners is a logical starting point in the planning process and can build longer-term working relationships.
- PhotoVoice, community asset mapping and grounded citizens' juries can help to engage people in local needs assessment.
- Top-down and bottom-up objectives can be accommodated within the same programme through parallel-tracking.

6 | Strategy selection

Health promotion theory includes a broad range of ideas and concepts, many of which have not been fully implemented or tested in practice. A major challenge in health promotion practice is how to apply the correct theory (the science) to the appropriate practice context (the art). Achieving both the 'art and science' of health promotion is possible through the selection of the best strategy for a particular programme context.

The 'art and science' of health promotion

> Applying the 'art and science' of health promotion does not guarantee a successful outcome but it does increase the chances of the programme being effective and sustainable.

Health promotion programmes cover a range of problems, partners, settings and cultural contexts, and in practice this may necessitate the use of more than one theory. On a day-to-day basis not all practitioners have the competencies to operate at multiple theoretical levels and are often constrained by time, finances and even the level of control that they have within a programme (Nutbeam et al., 2010).

Upstream and downstream

The terms upstream and downstream refer to the level of an intervention to positively impact on the health of people. At the individual (downstream) level, the intervention may be used to target people for a condition based on strategies such as screening for the early signs of diabetes. At the population (upstream) level, the intervention works to address the determinants of health which relate to the structural conditions under which people live: for example, policies to reduce sugary drinks in schools.

> The analogy is used of dragging drowning people from a flooded river (downstream) without going (upstream) to discover the reason why and to prevent the people from falling or being pushed into the river.

Downstream interventions are sometimes considered to be futile and short term. Contemporary practice in health promotion uses a holistic approach that identifies upstream socio-economic variables such as poverty and social injustice. It focuses on the 'causes of the causes' of the upstream variables that create poor health in the first instance. The resulting upstream causality thinking has yielded a discussion of attribution of effect that embraces the social determinants of health with a greatly diminished regard to downstream interventions seen as being individual-based and too focused on health education (McQueen and De Salazar, 2011).

Health promotion theory

Theory is systematically organised knowledge applicable in a relatively wide variety of circumstances devised to analyse, predict or otherwise explain the nature or behaviour of a specified set of phenomena (Van Ryn and Heany, 1992). Health promotion theory originates from the social and behavioural sciences drawing on knowledge from psychology, sociology, management, marketing, community development and the political sciences.

The weak evidence base of health promotion theory has resulted in the development of models for practice that seek to represent simplified versions of reality but that do not truly reflect the complexities (Naidoo and Wills, 2009). Practitioners often think in terms of the health-related 'problem' such as how to increase physical activity in the general population. A useful approach to select the best theory is to consider how it will address the health-related problem through, for example, communication and behaviour change, social change, empowerment or policy development (see table 6.1). This is then set within the overall purpose of enabling people to gain more control over their lives and to improve health.

Health promotion programmes sometimes have to operate at multiple levels to address the complex influences that contribute to inequalities in health. However, as no one model can be applied to fulfil the requirements of a comprehensive programme several theories would have to be utilised. For example, to encourage physical activity in children living in a deprived area would require an educational approach to raise awareness, a socio-environmental approach to change the physical environment to promote physical activity and an empowerment approach to address people's needs through local solutions (Gottwald and Goodman-Brown, 2012).

Table 6.1 Summary of health promotion theories and models

Programme purpose	Theories or models	Explanation
Communication and motivational strategies to achieve awareness-raising and behaviour change focused on the individual. Communication and motivational strategies to achieve awareness-raising and behaviour change focused on small groups.	• Health belief model • Reasoned action and planned behaviour change • Stages of change model • Social cognitive theory • Health literacy mode • Behaviour change theory • Social marketing theory	These theories use health education and the importance of self-belief in one's ability to change behaviour, the development of personal skills and the importance of perceived norms and social influences on the individual such as the role of family, friends and peer groups.
Community action for health.	• Community organisation and mobilisation theory • Diffusion of innovation theory • Empowerment theory	These theories provide opportunities for community-based intervention and empowerment, and for addressing the broader socio-economic determinants of health.
To influence the development and implementation of policy.	Theories for making and influencing healthy public policy	These theories provide a framework to intercede in the policy-making process, to lever and to change decisions.

> Health promotion models tend to be too theoretical and cannot be readily applied, or else offer little guidance to effective implementation in a complex environment.

From a practical perspective, it is useful to employ models and theories that use criteria similar to the purpose of the programme. These may include increased personal responsibility or autonomous choice; they might address the determinants of health or achieve a lifestyle and behavioural change. The programme can then employ the appropriate tools, methods and techniques that will best assist in the delivery of the activities necessary to achieve its purpose. Implicit in the selection of a strategy is the theory that explains how and why its different aspects are connected (Naidoo and Wills, 2009). When choosing a theory to best fit the programme it is useful to follow some simple questions. These will help to guide the selection of a strategy that is based on evidence, that is appropriate to the programme context and that is measurable:

- Is it simple to understand and logical?
- Does it match everyday observations of the problem?
- Has it been successfully used previously in a similar context?
- Is it supported by both scientific and anecdotal evidence of what works?
- Can it be justified in terms of the resources available?
- Can it be measured? (Glanz et al., 2008)

Health promotion approaches

Choosing a strategic approach

The strategic approach is usually pre-packaged and includes a description of an appropriate theory, model or approach, the partners or beneficiaries, the settings that they occupy, the channels of communication, and the tools that will be used to deliver services, training and resources. Health promotion approaches help to better understand the different ways of working in practice. The different approaches are historically based, sometimes contradictory, and without any one being dominant or sufficient to meet the requirements of present practice (Naidoo and Wills, 2009). The most commonly professionally recognised approaches include:

- the medical approach;
- the educational approach;
- the behavioural/lifestyle approach;
- the lifespan approach;
- the socio-environmental approach;
- the health inequalities agenda; and
- the ecological approach.

In practice, health promotion approaches largely determine the delivery and the evaluation criteria that are used in a programme. The development of these approaches in recent decades has resulted not only from the changes in our scientific understanding, but also from the growing pressure from individuals, groups and health social movements concerned with the determinants of health (Laverack, 2004).

The medical approach

The medical approach evolved as a result of scientific discoveries and technological advances in the 18th and 19th centuries leading to a greater understanding of the structure and functioning of the human body. The medical profession established itself in the dominant position and other health professions – including nursing, physiotherapy and, until recently, health promotion – soon modelled themselves on this approach to gain legitimacy. The medical approach is primarily concerned with the treatment of illness among high-risk individuals, those persons whose genetic predisposition, behaviour or personal history place them at statistically greater risk of disease. Despite the evolution of competing approaches it remains dominant within health bureaucracies because it has the advantage of focusing on the individual (Scriven, 2010). Health promotion programmes that use the medical approach focus on preventing an illness, disease or medical condition: for example, the promotion of immunisation to prevent the spread of measles. It does not focus on the structural causes of disease such as poverty and therefore conveniently allows the broader structural issues to be ignored. A growing body of new knowledge and pressure from health social movements has challenged the dominance of the medical approach, and this has led to a broadening of knowledge to include a variety of social, behavioural and lifestyle factors (Laverack, 2004). The medical approach, however, is still commonly used in health promotion programmes.

The educational approach

The educational approach helps individuals and groups to make an informed choice by using awareness-raising techniques. An informed choice is one that is based on relevant knowledge about a health behaviour and the perceived risk associated with a wrong choice, consistent with the decision-maker's values and behaviour (Dormandy et al., 2002).

> The educational approach recognises that knowledge alone is not enough to lead to behaviour change, which also requires a supportive environment.

Health promotion programmes that use the educational approach focus on the transfer of knowledge on a particular health issue: for example, information about the symptoms of diabetes. With this newly acquired information people can then make an informed decision about, for example, seeking further advice from a health professional. However, because of the complex social and cultural circumstances associated with behaviour change an individual may also choose not to make healthy choices or positive changes to their lifestyles, even if they have been well informed. In part, this is because making the healthy choice is not an easy option due to the lack of a supportive environment: for example, people wishing to do more physical activity do not have easy and affordable access to exercise facilities.

Fear appeals

The use of fear appeals are sometimes implemented in the educational approach: for example, using graphic images of cancer to dissuade people from smoking. A fear appeal involves threatening the target audience with harmful outcomes for starting or continuing a particular high-risk behaviour. Fear appeals can sometimes be effective when they are combined with an easy solution to rectify the harmful high-risk behaviour. However, campaigns rarely include the necessary skills development that is also needed to resolve the high-risk behaviour and instead rely on the individual or on other services, including the commercial sector, to provide supportive services and products (Corcoran, 2013). Appeals designed to invoke guilt and shame can also confuse or increase the level of perceived fear within the targeted population. One study, for example, showed that negative appeals in a social marketing campaign designed to increase compliance with income-reporting requirements were more likely to invoke self-protection and inaction rather than an active response such as volunteering to comply (Brennan and Binney, 2010). In another study involving 840 young adults, the use of fear appeals changed participants' beliefs and intentions about distractions caused by four unsafe driving behaviours. After viewing two fear appeals, participants reported increased intentions of actually engaging in the unsafe behaviours, especially the males, and aroused only low-to-moderate levels of fear in the young adults. The study concluded that the fear appeal was not effective enough in reaching young adults on the issue of safe driving (Lennon et al., 2010).

The behavioural/lifestyle approach

The behavioural/lifestyle approach became increasingly central to health promotion in the late 1970s through campaigns around smoking, alcohol abuse and physical inactivity. Many practitioners had found that health education campaigns alone, a key strategy in the lifestyle approach, did not succeed in changing behaviour and proved difficult to link to subsequent changes in health and wellbeing. In theory, the approach does not view behaviour as an isolated action but recognises how it is influenced and conditioned by a complex interplay of other factors. However, in practice the lifestyle approach continues to place a strong emphasis on the responsibility of the individual and the importance of education.

Despite the modest evidence for the success of the behavioural/ lifestyle approach it remains a popular option for health promotion practice. Programmes using this approach focus on providing people with the knowledge and skills that are necessary for them to adopt a healthier lifestyle or behaviour: for example, to use condoms for safer sex. The approach remains popular because it offers the simple logic of behaviour change through education and motivational strategies that can be easily delivered in a programme context.

The lifespan approach

The lifespan approach to health promotion focuses on how our needs and bodies change throughout our lives. The approach is based on providing appropriate interventions at the different stages of a person's lifespan to promote health and wellbeing (Hubley and Copeman, 2013).

Age in years is most often used in the lifespan approach although there is some overlap between the different stages in health promotion programmes. It is therefore important to carefully identify which age groups the interventions will focus on; this, in part, will also be determined by the demographics of the target population. Within the specific age groups it is then necessary to identify the health promotion needs and the strategies that can be used most effectively. This is because people are faced with different risk factors and have access to different resources in their lifespan.

A lifespan approach for health promotion would typically use the following stages:

- From pre-conception to birth the health of the baby is affected by the nutrition and health of the mother. Health promotion interventions would include policy promotion for folic acid to reduce the risk of spina bifida, education programmes to warn about the risks of drinking during pregnancy and health literacy to promote breastfeeding.
- The first years of life (0–4 years) are a period of rapid physical and psychological development, and health promotion interventions would include promoting social and mental stimulation, nutrition and support to parents.
- The pre-pubescent child (aged 5–9 years) is exposed to a much wider circle of contacts and may be the subject of bullying and abuse. Health promotion interventions for this age are most often channelled through the school setting as well as through social clubs and interest groups.

- The pubescent and adolescent (10–17 years) school age marks major physical changes as well as a social dimension in which there is a transition from childhood to adulthood. Health promotion places more responsibility on the individual for their own behaviour related to, for example, substance abuse and sex education.
- In many cultures a young person (18–24 years) legally and socially becomes an adult around 18 years of age. However, it is also a confusing time in which many pressures are placed on the young person, such as employment or continued education, and can lead to stress in their lives. Health promotion interventions may target substance abuse, isolation and mental illnesses through, for example, peer education and social media.
- Middle adulthood (25–49 years) is a time for establishing a pattern in life, raising a family and dealing with a breakdown in relationships. The role of health promotion is to ensure that people are supported on a range of health and parenting issues, often through a variety of services such as clinical settings, health workers and child care services.
- Older adulthood (50–69 years) is the start of a transition to being elderly and a period when people can suffer from chronic diseases such as cancers and heart disease. The emphasis is on maintaining a healthy lifestyle and coping with life-changing experiences such as bereavements and the menopause.
- It is important to distinguish between the 'well old' and the 'frail old' among the elderly (70 years onwards), as it is in the latter that the elderly person will need special attention from health promotion interventions. Key concerns are isolation, disability, osteoporosis, abuse and coping with poverty, such as keeping warm in winter and having a balanced diet (Hubley and Copeman, 2013).

The socio-environmental approach

The medical, educational, behavioural/lifestyle and lifespan approaches have served an important role in the development of health promotion but do not fully recognise the broad structural issues which powerfully influence health. Health social movements challenged the notion of the medical and behavioural/lifestyle approaches and a new, emancipatory discourse on health promotion began to form, one more concerned with social justice than with individual behaviour change. The socio-environmental approach focuses on society and how it can change in order to promote people's health by addressing their social and environmental conditions. The socio-environmental approach also addresses the distribution of resources and engaging with people to influence policy decisions. Collective empowerment is a central strategy to enable people to have more of a 'voice' about their health and health care and also to be able to take action if this does not meet their needs and expectations. The value of empowerment is that it enables people to become better organised and mobilised, to network and to move towards social and political action.

The health inequalities agenda

Health inequity is shaped by deep social structures and processes and can be enhanced by social norms and government policies that tolerate or actually promote the unfair distribution of and access to power, wealth and social resources (WHO, 2008). A health inequity is a difference (an inequality) in health that is significant in the number of people affected, preventable through policy or another intervention and not an effect of freely chosen risk. The inequalities in everyday living include unequal access to health care and education, conditions of work and the limited opportunities to lead a healthy life. This unequal distribution is the result of a combination of poor social policies and programmes, unfair economic arrangements and unjust governance. People who, for example, have high-risk lifestyles or poor living conditions are typically influenced more by economic and political policies, suffer greater health inequalities and consequently have more disease and premature death, and less wellbeing (Wilkinson, 2003).

Lifestyle drift

Health promotion programmes sometimes start with a commitment to address the health inequalities agenda only to 'drift' inevitably to much narrower lifestyle interventions. This political trend has been termed the 'lifestyle drift' and can be illustrated by the 'Swap it, don't stop it' campaign in Australia. The main character of the campaign is 'Eric', a blue balloon type figure, who urges others to swap unhealthy aspects of their lifestyle, such as poor eating habits and physical inactivity, for healthier lifestyle habits. However, the changes necessary for 'Eric' to lead a healthier life actually require a change in the structures in which he lives, such as an affordable healthy diet and a safe neighbourhood: structural changes conveniently ignored by the government (Baum, 2011), which instead focused on targeting a modification of individual 'unhealthy' lifestyles.

The ecological approach

The ecological approach is based in part upon an understanding of human ecology as the interaction of culture with the environment. The approach encompasses culture and the biosphere, which ultimately is our living planet. Health is understood in its holistic sense, so the health of the individual is at the centre of the ecosystem and has body, mind and spiritual dimensions. The approach has system levels extending outwards from the individual representing the family, the community and its built environment, and the wider society and natural environment, exemplified by culture and biosphere. The approach integrates the social sciences with the natural sciences and indicates that the 'healthcare' system is only one determinant of health. The ecological approach makes it clear that no single strategy and no effort focused on only one aspect of the determinants of health can be wholly successful (Hancock, 1993).

> The practitioner must be prepared to operate at multiple theoretical levels and with competing models and approaches in order to select the best fit to a particular programme.

Identifying your partners

Within a programme context there is always some relationship between the practitioners and the range of people with whom they work to improve or maintain their health. Different terms are used to describe these people, including the primary stakeholders, the beneficiaries, the target audience or the partners with whom the services, information and resources are shared through the programme. The beneficiaries are those people who are ultimately affected and at whom the programme is usually targeted. Other partners act as an intermediary in the delivery of the programme: for example, health promotion agencies and the practitioners that they employ. I have used the term 'partners' to cover the different stakeholders, beneficiaries and target audiences in health promotion programmes. The partners include adults and adolescents of both sexes from different socio-economic and cultural groups and who occupy different settings (Laverack, 2009). These partners are identified during the planning phase and may be involved in the programme as individuals, as social groups, as a 'community of interest' or as a geographical community, or included as part of a broader approach within civil society.

The partners are identified according to the requirements of the programme purpose often using a stratification of categories including age, gender, marital status, ethnicity and socio-economic background. A lifespan approach to health promotion, for example, typically uses age in years to target the programme partners, whereas a lifestyle approach would target individuals involved in high-risk behaviours. Health promotion may also target marginalised groups that exist on the fringes of a society and from where they can become excluded from access to services thus leading to poorer health.

Paying attention to marginalisation

> Marginalisation is a process by which an individual or a group is denied access to, or positions of, economic, religious and political power within a society (Marshall, 1998).

The circumstances of marginalisation – including poverty, discrimination and racism – can contribute to low self-esteem and to the exclusion from health promotion programmes. In practical terms, marginalised groups are considered to be those that are most in need, are not able to meet their own needs, have a limited access to resources, are powerless or exist largely outside dominant social power structures. The marginalised include people of a low socio-economic status but can also be groups excluded because of their gender, age, ethnicity, (dis)ability and/or sexual preference.

Migrants are an example of marginalised groups. Migration – either in terms of internal migration, where no national boundaries are crossed, or international migration, where people move to another place across national boundaries – occurs for a variety of reasons. For example, people may leave their home to look for better economic opportunities, because of oppressive political circumstances, to be with family, for education or because they are forced to move. Migration is not always intended to be permanent, and many people may wish to return to their home country at some stage in the future (MacPherson and Gushulak, 2004). When living in a new country many migrants are faced with restricted legal rights; a poor understanding of the local language, culture and systems; different religious beliefs; and a low income. This can lead to feelings of alienation and of being placed in a more vulnerable position of poor physical and mental health (Laverack, 2009).

Health promotion settings

> A setting is a place or social context in which people engage in daily activities and in which environmental, organisational and personal factors interact to affect health and wellbeing (WHO, 1998).

Programme partners occupy a setting in which they engage in their daily activities of work and recreation. It may have physical boundaries and include a range of people with defined roles, an organisational structure or a spatial location. Settings can be used to promote health by reaching people who occupy them and who use them to gain access to services or through changing the physical and policy environment. A settings approach to health promotion aims to make systematic changes to the whole environment and not just use it as a channel through which to gain access to and to educate people (Naidoo and Wills, 2009). However, the complexity of the settings approach has made the evaluation of its effectiveness problematic, confounded by the lack of a credible theoretical framework that explains how and why the approach functions (WHO, 1998). Settings that are commonly used in health promotion programmes include health promoting hospitals, schools, workplaces and cities.

Health promoting hospitals

A health promoting hospital does not only provide high-quality medical and nursing services, but also develops a corporate identity that embraces the aims of health promotion, and develops a health promoting organisational structure, culture and physical environment. Health promoting hospitals take a holistic approach to promote the health of their patients, their staff, and the population within the community in which they are located.

Health promoting schools

Health promoting schools are characterised as constantly strengthening their capacity as a healthy setting for living, learning and working. A health promoting school engages health and education officials, teachers, unions, students, parents, health providers and community leaders. A healthy environment is provided through health education and health services, school/community programmes, and physical education, recreation and counselling. The school implements policies and practices that respect an individual's wellbeing and dignity as well as the health of school personnel, families and community members.

Health promoting workplaces

In the 1990s, workplace health promotion re-oriented to be more holistic and to address both individual risk factors and broader organisational and environmental issues. For example, instead of using the workplace as a convenient location to change individual behaviours, workplace health promotion involved both workers and management collectively, endeavouring to change the workplace into a health promoting setting (Chu et al., 2000). The World Health Organization has called for the development of a comprehensive approach towards the promotion of the health of all working populations. This approach is based upon four fundamental complementary principles: health promotion, occupational health and safety, human resource management, and sustainable development. Fundamental to this approach are multi-sectoral partnerships and the involvement and cooperation of the key actors (WHO, 1997).

Healthy cities

A healthy city is continually creating and improving physical and social environments and expanding community resources which enable people to mutually support each other (WHO, 1998). The healthy city programme is a long-term international initiative that aims to place health high on the agendas of decision-makers and to promote comprehensive local strategies for health protection and sustainable development. The healthy city concept depends on a commitment to improve a city's environs and a willingness to create the necessary connections in political, economic, and social arenas. It includes community participation and empowerment, and inter-sectoral partnerships, and is evolving to encompass other forms of settlement including healthy villages and municipalities.

Key points of the chapter

- The practitioner must be prepared to operate at multiple theoretical levels with competing models and approaches to select the best fit to a particular programme.
- Applying the 'art and science' of health promotion does not guarantee a successful outcome but it does increase the chances of the programme being effective and sustainable.
- It is important that practitioners are sensitive to the circumstances that can affect the participation of marginalised groups in programmes.
- A settings approach offers a useful channel through which to access and educate people and also to make changes to the whole environment.

7 Strategy implementation for individuals and groups

The purpose of strategy implementation is to deliver information, resources and services that improve health and enable people to gain more control over their lives. Individual action is a crucial first step towards acquiring greater control, and once this process has begun people can better participate in groups and communities that share their needs and concerns. Ultimately, it is through collective, rather than individual, action that people can address the broader causes of health inequality. To understand how practitioners can assist individuals and groups this chapter discusses different strategies that can be used in health promotion programmes.

Working with individuals

Helping individuals to gain more control over their lives and health begins by increasing their knowledge, by developing their skills and, most importantly, by creating a dialogue to help them to identify personal issues and potential solutions. Methods that can be used during the strategy implementation to achieve awareness-raising and skills development when working at an individual level include one-to-one communication (including counselling), peer education and using a client-centred approach.

One-to-one communication

Communication can be individually focused on a basis of one (the practitioner) to one (the partner): for example, a doctor talking to a patient. One-to-one communication is important because this allows a dialogue to develop between the partner and the practitioner. The dialogue is based on a sharing of knowledge and experiences in a two-way communication that is necessary to help individuals to better retain information, to clarify personal issues and to develop skills and coping strategies.

Effective one-to-one communication should follow a simple procedure of listening, giving advice, and obtaining and providing feedback, normally directed by the practitioner. Listening is an active process focusing on what the individual is saying and if necessary helping the speaker to express his/her feelings or to give an opinion on an issue. When giving advice the practitioner is exerting his/her expert power whilst the partner accepts an obligation to comply with the advice. This is sometimes a necessary communication style when, for example, helping someone understand a sensitive issue such as the result of a medical test (Hubley and Copeman, 2013). Obtaining and giving feedback enables the practitioner to clarify what the partner really needs and that they have understood previous communication and retained skills. This may mean obtaining feedback based on specific information using closed questions that require short factual (yes/no) answers or based on an open form of questioning to provide fuller answers. Giving feedback is important for the achievement of effective communication, and in particular positive feedback reinforces the partner's knowledge level.

Counselling

Counselling is a form of one-to-one communication and an interaction in which someone seeks to explore, understand or resolve a problem. The counselling occurs when a person consults someone else regarding a problem that is preventing them from living their lives in a way that they would wish to do so (McLeod and McLeod, 2011). Counselling can involve people working in any kind of helping or managing, or in a facilitative role including in social work and health education. Counsellors help others explore and understand their worlds and so discover better ways of thinking and living. This can be delivered through a number of methods including interpersonal communication, interviewing and shared decision-making.

A common factor in counselling situations is that the client is emotionally distressed or in a negative state of mind about something. This is when professional counselling and therapy skills are required beyond the competencies of most health promoters. Whilst the boundaries are not always clear, therapy can be used in a more clinical context, whilst counselling tends to have a more social focus. A critical variable in the style of counselling used is the extent to which the solutions to problems are provided by the counsellor or by the client. This leads to two different roles for the counsellor: problem-solver and facilitator (Dryden and Feltham, 1993).

Peer education

Peer education is an approach in which people are supported to promote health-enhancing change among their peers. Rather than health professionals educating members of the public, laypeople are felt to be in the best position to encourage healthy behaviour with each other. Peer education has become very popular in the field of HIV prevention, especially involving young people, sex workers, men who have sex with men, and intravenous drug users. Peer education is also associated with efforts to prevent tobacco, drug or alcohol use among young people, teenage pregnancy and homelessness. Peer education is usually initiated by practitioners who recruit members of the 'target' community to serve as educators. Peer educators are typically about the same age as the group with whom they are working. The recruited peer educators are trained in relevant communication skills and then engage their peers, seeking to promote health-enhancing behaviour change. The intention is that familiar people, giving locally relevant and meaningful suggestions, in the same language will be more likely to promote health. They may work alongside the health promoter, run educational activities on their own, or take the lead in organising and implementing activities (Robertson et al., 2010).

'Befriending' offers supportive, reliable relationships through peers for people who would otherwise be socially isolated. It is an internationally recognised approach, and in the UK befriending projects organise effective support for children and young people, families, people with mental illhealth, people with learning disabilities and older people. However, peer education interventions can have a high attrition rate as volunteers may leave the programme for personal reasons and financial constraints. Befriending work can be emotionally demanding, and volunteers do sometimes get depressed and leave even though they can speak to one another or to a practitioner about their problems: for example, a befriending coordinator can act as a mentor to newly recruited peer educators (Falkirk Council/HealthProm, 2013).

The evidence on peer education is mixed, seemingly working in some contexts but not in others. Peer education should therefore be seen as a strategy that can be used alongside other strategies in a broader health promotion approach: for example, it has been used effectively to complement skills-based health education on condom promotion and for youth-friendly health services (UNICEF, 2013). Peer education should not be seen as a cheap strategy option, because it requires a significant commitment for training and the provision of resources to the peer educators.

The client-centred approach

Decision-making at an individual level can be a useful way to help an individual gain more control over health issues in their life. However, barriers and constraints can make this difficult to achieve and therefore a client-centred approach can be used to help promote the basic principles of individual responsibility. The client-centred approach focuses on the perspective of the individual to help them to identify and to address their own health issues. The client is encouraged to share their concerns, feelings and opinions, usually facilitated by the practitioner using a 'client-centred' technique such as the patient-centred clinical method (Stewart et al., 2003). A more equal relationship is then created, one in which the practitioner uses their knowledge to allow the patient to make informed decisions about their treatment and recovery.

The patient-centred clinical method

The patient-centred clinical method applies the principles of individual empowerment in a practitioner–patient relationship as follows:

1 The illness and the patient's experience of being ill are explored at the same time.
2 Understanding the person as a whole places the illness into context by considering how the illness affects the person, how the person interacts with their immediate environment, and how the wider environment influences this interaction.
3 The patient and doctor reach a mutual understanding on the nature of the illness, its causes and its goals for management, and who is responsible for what.
4 The desirability and applicability to undertake broader health promoting and illness-prevention tasks are explored: for example, providing the patient with information or skills about how they can dress their own wound at home.
5 A better understanding of the patient–doctor relationship is thus gained in order to enhance it: for example, placing a value on the contribution being made by both sides and forming a 'partnership' to address the illness rather than a traditional paternalistic approach.
6 A realistic assessment is made of what can be done to help the patient given, for example, constraints in understanding, time and skill level (Stewart et al., 2003).

Giving the patient more control over decisions can have real benefits, as demonstrated in one study (Bassett and Prapavessis, 2007) on physical therapy for ankle sprains. The study showed that the home-based groups had similar outcome scores for post-treatment ankle function, adherence and motivation to a standard physical-therapy intervention. However, the home-based group had significantly better attendance at clinic appointments and a better physical-therapy completion rate. Patients were helped to set goals and to develop personal action plans to complete the therapy, as well as receiving education and skills training on the treatment, such as strapping techniques. Giving the patient more control can be a complicated issue that is not appropriate for all situations or people, but under the right conditions, as this study showed, it can offer the practitioner the opportunity to work in a more empowering way.

Dealing with powerlessness

Some people simply do not want to be involved in health promotion programmes. People, especially if they have lived in oppressive or powerless circumstances, may feel that they do not have the right or do not possess the ability to take more control over their health. These individuals can internalise the sense of lack of control in their lives to create a psychological barrier to self-help. Powerlessness, or the absence of power, whether imagined or real, is a concept with the expectancy that their behaviour cannot determine the outcomes they seek. Powerlessness combines an attitude of self-blame, a sense of generalised distrust, a feeling of alienation from resources, an experience of disenfranchisement and economic vulnerability, and a sense of hopelessness in political struggle (Freire, 2005).

Learned helplessness is the condition of learning to behave in a powerless way, failing to respond even though there are opportunities to help oneself. Learned helplessness may result from a perceived absence of control over the outcome of a situation such as unemployment, poverty or homelessness. People think that these are unalterable features of what they take to be reality. Learned helplessness can contribute to poor health when people, for example, neglect exercise and medical treatment, and the more people perceive events as uncontrollable, the more stress they experience. It has been shown, for example, that this has corresponding symptoms in poor mental health (Seligman, 1990). Powerlessness can therefore be a result of the passive acceptance of oppressive norms that can be exacerbated by public policy that cuts pay and jobs, freezes benefits and welfare payments, and reduces opportunities for education and the maintenance of a supportive infrastructure (Nathanson and Hopper, 2010).

Do people have a right not to become empowered? What must be remembered is that power cannot be given but people must gain it for themselves, and the right to be empowered rests with the individual and not with the practitioner. Learned optimism is contrasted with learned helplessness by people consciously challenging any negative aspects in their lives, and can be enhanced through therapy, critical education and counselling. People can be helped to fight against the perception that events are uncontrollable by increasing their awareness of previous experiences, when they were able to effect a desired outcome (Seligman, 1990).

> The role of the practitioner in helping others to overcome powerlessness is to enable them to take greater responsibility and control over their health and lives.

People who do not want the responsibility of making decisions or have a fear of the regret of making a misjudgement can delegate this authority to another person in whom they have some trust. Other individuals – for example, the very young, the very old or people with an addiction – may not have the ability to sufficiently organise and mobilise themselves collectively. For those people who cannot or who refuse to take responsibility then the practitioner may have to intervene and resort to a more paternalistic approach. In practice, health policy and legislation are used in this way to prevent the spread of an infectious disease, or place an individual into care (even against their wishes) to ensure the wellbeing of themselves and of others.

Working with groups

Working with groups is an important part of health promotion because this is often the point at which individuals are able to progress onto collective action. Small groups allow people to become better organised and mobilised towards addressing their health needs. Working with groups also provides an opportunity for the practitioner to assist others to develop stronger social links and skills, and to raise the resources necessary to support their actions. Small groups often begin with a focus on the immediate needs of their members, but with sufficient capacity-building this focus can broaden to include the causes of inequality and social injustice.

Methods that can be used to achieve stronger social support and skills development in small groups include self-help, health literacy and strategies for collective decision-making.

Self-help groups

> Self-help groups organise around a specific issue, are inward looking, and aim to help others to find solutions, provide support or to develop skills to address a variety of problems.

Self-help is a self-guided improvement that often utilises support groups, either face to face or through the Internet, to provide friendship, emotional support, information and a greater sense of belonging (Farris-Kurtz, 1997). People go to self-help groups for a variety of reasons: some simply want information and will then move on, whilst others may want to make sense of what is happening to them by sharing their experiences with those who have been through something similar. Members of the group have a shared knowledge and interest in the problem, are supportive of one another and often manage activities by themselves. Mutual support is a common technique used in self-help groups by which people voluntarily come together to talk and to help each other to address common problems. Self-help groups can therefore bring people together to help them to address issues which they feel are relevant to their health, including disability, smoking cessation, weight loss, addiction and depression. By using a facilitated dialogue the self-help group can also be an important starting point for promoting coping skills, positive behaviour change and various therapies for recovery from long-term health issues.

The challenge is to enable individuals to move beyond addressing personal issues, to work with others who share the same concerns to achieve longer-lasting changes.

In an empowering approach, a key challenge when working with self-help groups is to enable individuals to move forward to work with others who share the same concerns and with whom they can achieve broader and longer-lasting changes. Self-help groups often have limited resources, and because of their small size they can be absorbed by a broader government agenda unless they are able to develop into a larger organisation (Allsop et al., 2004). Needs assessment skills, for example, are necessary to be able to identify the common problems of their members, solutions to the problems, and actions to resolve the problems (see chapter 5). Other key characteristics of better organisation include meeting on a regular basis, a structure (chairperson, secretary, core members), keeping records and financial accounts and the ability to identify and resolve conflicts quickly (Jones and Laverack, 2003).

One example of an issue where self-help groups have proved useful is female genital cutting (FGC), which comprises all procedures involving partial or total removal of the external female genitalia or other injury to the female genital organs whether for cultural, religious or non-therapeutic reasons. Self-help services are offered, for example, to refugees to cope with the distress of this experience. The purpose is to motivate an understanding that these traditional practices are harmful to the health of girls and women, and, therefore, violations of their human rights and not in accordance with their religious and cultural values (Reaves, 2007). The focus of the self-help group gradually changes to an outward-looking orientation, including advocacy work on the issue of FGC. This is further advanced through interagency groups of health and government organisations that can assist in the lobbying efforts of the women themselves. Thus the health promotion programme can help the self-help group to grow and to create community-led action to change, for example, policy and legislation in regard to FGC with long-lasting benefits for all women.

Health promoters can help individuals to advance into organisations that address their needs at a broader level through networking and capacity-building, and by increasing their level of critical consciousness (chapter 8). A first step towards achieving these goals is the development of personal skills – for example, through health literacy, and strategies for collective decision-making – and this is discussed next.

Health literacy

> Health literacy is more than just the transmission of information and is focused on skills development so as to help others to make informed decisions that will allow them to exert greater control on their lives and health (Renkert and Nutbeam, 2001).

Health literacy is a repackaging of the relationship between health education and empowerment. Health literacy grew out of the realisation that interventions that relied heavily on information towards behaviour change failed to achieve substantial results (Nutbeam, 2000). The value of health literacy is as a tool to help practitioners increase the knowledge, skills and the critical awareness of individual partners. Health literacy involves cognitive and social skills which determine the motivation and ability of individuals to gain access to, understand and use information in ways that promote and maintain good health (WHO, 1998).

Three levels of health literacy

Health literacy is often dependent on the level of basic literacy in the community – that is, the ability to read and write in everyday life – and what this enables people to do. Health literacy therefore has three levels that can take into account the different levels of ability in a community:

1 Basic/functional literacy: sufficient basic skills in reading and writing to be able to function effectively in everyday situations, broadly compatible with the narrow definition.
2 Communicative/interactive literacy: more advanced cognitive and literacy skills which, together with social skills, can be used to actively participate in everyday activities, to extract information and derive meaning from different forms of communication, and to apply new information to changing circumstances.
3 Critical literacy: more advanced cognitive skills which, together with social skills, can be applied to critically analyse information, and to use this information to exert greater control over life events and situations (Nutbeam, 2000).

The challenge is to use advanced methods of health education aimed at achieving critical health literacy rather than basic or functional health literacy.

Health literacy has been specifically developed within health promotion to allow the practitioner to focus on the development of life skills which enable individuals to deal effectively with the challenges of everyday life. Life skills consist of personal, inter-personal, cognitive and physical skills which enable people to control their lives and to produce change in their environment (WHO, 1998).

Life skills for health promotion

Life skills are described as a key action area for health promotion through decision-making and problem-solving, creative and critical thinking, self-awareness, communication skills and strategies to cope with emotions (WHO, 1986). In practice these translate into everyday personal skills such as smoking cessation, breastfeeding, hand-washing, coping with stress and coping with bullying.

An example of the potential use of health literacy is in antenatal classes to provide women with the cognitive and social skills they need to maintain their health and that of their children. Women attending antenatal classes are often highly motivated and literate. But antenatal classes are sometimes constrained by time, and the natural curiosity and anxiety of the women makes it difficult to transfer all the necessary information and skills. Classes therefore focus on the transfer of factual information rather than on decision-making skills for childbirth and parenting, which can occupy more time. Decision-making can be empowering and is central to the use of health literacy techniques that focus on enabling women to make informed choices. In this way the entire content of the antenatal class would not have to be delivered, reducing the time needed for teaching and providing more time to allow the mothers to ask questions and to discuss issues (Renkert and Nutbeam, 2001).

> Health literacy offers an advanced educational approach that enables people to take action to address their problems.

Strategies for collective decision-making

Decision-making, even at a group level, can be a complex procedure but can also be an empowering experience for people in regard to a range of health choices. A practical and field-tested approach to promote the basic principles of collective decision-making is outlined below.

Ranking key choices

Group members first make a ranked list of the key choices covering their particular collective health concern. The practitioner can help by providing specific technical information to answer any questions about the issue. The ranking must come from the individuals in the group without being led by the practitioner. If the number of ranked choices is large, the practitioner can assist the individuals to produce a more prioritised list. For example, a ranked list for health choices in regard to becoming healthier might include:

1 To stop smoking in the next six months.
2 To do more exercise.
3 To lose weight.
4 To eat more healthily.

A ranking of the different choices is in itself insufficient to empower others who must also have the ability to transform this information into decisions and actions. This is achieved through developing a decision-making matrix for positive changes in the prioritised areas using:

- decisions on the key actions to be taken;
- decisions on the key activities for each action taken; and
- the identification of resources.

Ranking is a simple exercise to 'unpack' the issues that influence people's health into its different elements so that they can be further analysed and addressed.

Decisions on the key actions to be taken

The group is next asked to decide on how the situation can be improved for each of its prioritised choices. The purpose is firstly to identify the most feasible actions that will improve the present situation and then to provide a lead-in to a more detailed strategy. This information is placed in column 2 of the matrix in figure 7.1. Taking the first ranked health choice (to stop smoking in the next 6 months), the decisions on the key actions to be taken might include:

Priority	Key decisions	Key activities	Resources
To stop smoking in the next 6 months.	To remove all cigarettes from the home and workplace. To attend motivation classes to help to stop smoking. To use a substitute for smoking such as chewing gum or nicotine patches.	Collect all cigarettes in house and dispose. Do not purchase any more cigarettes. Identify local classes. Make time to attend one class per week. Identify a friend to attend initial classes for support. Discuss best alternative products with a doctor or pharmacist. Make an appointment to speak with a doctor in the next 7 days. Buy product from pharmacy. Take on a prescribed basis for the next 3 months.	The availability of a local self-motivation class. Money to pay for classes and time to attend them. Access to a pharmacy or practitioner to discuss the best choices for a smoking substitute. Money to purchase substitute products.

Figure 7.1 The decision-making matrix

- To remove all cigarettes from the home and workplace.
- To attend motivation classes to help to stop smoking.
- To use a substitute for smoking such as chewing gum or nicotine patches.

Decisions on the key activities for each action taken

The group is then asked to consider in practice the most feasible actions that can be carried out. In particular, they are asked to identify specific activities, to sequence activities in order to make an improvement and to set a realistic timeframe including any significant targets. These are placed in column 3 of the matrix. The activities to implement the identified actions to stop smoking might include the following:

- Collect all cigarettes in house and dispose.
- Do not purchase any more cigarettes.
- Identify local classes. Make time to attend one class per week. Identify a friend to attend initial classes for support.
- Discuss best alternative products with a doctor or pharmacist. Make an appointment to speak with a doctor in the next 7 days.
- Buy product from pharmacy. Take on a prescribed basis for the next 3 months.

Identification of resources

The group next identify the resources that are necessary to implement the actions in column 3. The practitioner can help them to map the necessary resources – for example, information, finances and emotional support – that are necessary to undertake the actions. The resources to help stop smoking might include:

- The availability of a local self-motivation class.
- Money to pay for classes and time to attend them.
- Access to a pharmacy or practitioner to discuss the best choices for a smoking substitute.
- Money to purchase substitute products.

The decision-making matrix

The strategy for decision-making can be represented by using a simplified matrix in which the ranking is placed in the left-hand column followed by sequential columns for:

1 prioritising the key health issues;
2 decisions on the key actions to be taken;
3 decisions on the key activities for each action taken; and
4 the identification of resources.

The matrix provides a summary of the decisions and actions to be undertaken and can be the basis for an 'informal contract' between the practitioner and the group. It identifies specific tasks or responsibilities usually set against a timeframe based on the period identified as being realistic: for example, to stop smoking, this was given as 6 months. It also identifies the resources or assistance that will be required to fulfil these tasks and responsibilities, within the agreed timeframe.

The group members have a shared knowledge and interest in smoking cessation and can support one another to achieve the goals that they have collectively agreed upon. The role of the practitioner is to facilitate this by helping individual members overcome barriers and by ensuring that the group meets on a regular basis to assess individual progress.

Key points of the chapter

- Individual action is a crucial first step towards acquiring greater control.
- Working with groups is important because this is the point at which individuals are better able to progress onto collective action.
- Power cannot be given but people must gain it for themselves.
- The right to be empowered rests with the individual and not with the practitioner.
- The challenge is to enable individuals to move beyond addressing personal issues, to work with others who share the same concerns to achieve longer-lasting changes.
- The role of the practitioner in helping others to overcome powerlessness is to enable them to take greater responsibility and control over their health and lives.

8 | Strategy implementation for communities

A key aspect of health promotion work is helping communities to identify their needs, to find a 'voice' to express their needs and to gain access to information, resources and services. This is especially important for the marginalised in society, including low-income communities, newly arrived migrants and resettlement neighbourhoods. Community-based interventions can work in the long term to help people to address health inequalities and in the short term to gain better access to health and social care services (South et al., 2013).

Working with communities

What is a 'community'?

Traditionally, a 'community' has been viewed as a place where people live: for example, a neighbourhood or a village. However, these are often just an aggregate of non-connected people. Communities also involve social interactions that are dynamic and bind people into relationships based on their shared needs (Laverack 2004). As a working 'rule of thumb' a community will occupy a spatial dimension – that is, a place or locale – and a non-spatial dimension that involves relationships between people. Within the geographic dimensions of a community, multiple non-spatial communities often exist, and individuals may belong to several different interest groups. Interest groups exist as a legitimate means by which individuals are organised around a variety of social activities (for example, sports events) or to address a shared concern (for example, the lack of public transport) (Zakus and Lysack, 1998). However, the diversity of interests within a community can sometimes create problems, and practitioners try to avoid the establishment of a dominant minority that can dictate issues based only on their concerns and not on those of the majority.

> Practitioners need to carefully consider if the representatives of a community are supported by its members and that they are not just acting out of self-interest.

What is 'civil society'?

Civil society goes beyond the concept of a 'community' to include people in both their social and professional contexts, including the totality of voluntary, civic and social organisations, which together form the basis of a functioning society. Civil society is important because it stresses the need for a developed level of public and political participation, both central to health promotion. Civil society works through people who create groups, organisations, communities and movements to address shared needs. Civil societies are populated by organisations such as registered charities, non-governmental organisations (NGOs), community groups, women's organisations, faith-based organisations, trade unions, self-help groups, social movements, and activist and advocacy groups (Laverack, 2013a: 19).

Health promoters can use a variety of methods to work better with communities, and these include improving the level of critical consciousness, building stronger partnerships, strengthening networks and building community capacity.

Improving the level of critical consciousness

Critical consciousness can be described as the ability to reflect on the assumptions underlying our actions and to contemplate better ways of living (Goodman et al., 1998).

Communities cannot intentionally empower themselves without having an understanding of the underlying causes of their powerlessness. This may occur from within the community, often developing slowly and organically. Alternatively, it can occur through an intervention that promotes a process of discussion, reflection and action. This process is called 'critical consciousness' or 'conscientisation' and involves learning using 'empowerment education' as developed by Paulo Freire (Freire, 2005). To Freire, the central premise was that education is not neutral but is influenced by the context of one's life. The purpose of education is liberation in which people become the subjects of their own learning, involving critical reflection and an analysis of their personal circumstances (Wallerstein and Bernstein, 1988). To achieve this, Freire proposed a group-dialogue approach to share ideas and experiences and to promote critical thinking by posing problems to allow people to uncover the root causes of their powerlessness. Once critically aware, people can then plan more effective actions to change their circumstances. Critical consciousness works by gradually understanding the causes of powerlessness and by developing realistic actions to begin to resolve the conditions that created them in the first place (Nutbeam, 2000).

A practical application of critical consciousness is through Photo-Voice (see chapter 5): for example, to help newcomer communities in Toronto, Canada.

Helping to improve the critical consciousness of newcomer communities

In an inner-city area of Toronto, PhotoVoice has been used to provide images of community issues, with a camera, by people living in new-comer communities. An account was then created to explain what was important in the pictures using these people's own words. The images were displayed at an exposition, and recommendations were made to the city authorities regarding bicycle theft due to improperly main-tained bicycle racks, which was identified as a common problem by the newcomer community. Since cycling is the main mode of transport for many residents, safe bicycle storage is a daily stressor for many people. The community worked with the city authorities to take an inventory of all bicycle racks, arrange the removal of broken bicycles from exis-ting racks and install new racks in the neighbourhood. The decision of the city authorities to remove broken and abandoned bicycles from the neighbourhood was as a direct result of the critical-consciousness approach (Haque and Eng, 2011).

Building stronger partnerships

Partnerships demonstrate the ability to develop relationships with dif-ferent organisations, to collaborate and to promote cooperation among its members. Partnerships are advantageous for working with commu-nities because they create shared values and collective goals, lead to the dissemination of information, reduce feelings of isolation and help with problem-solving (Kumpfer et al., 1993). Partnerships have become a popular theme in health promotion, but it is essential that they are participatory so that government organisations do not merely consult with the community but, rather, that people are involved in a two-way process of decision-making.

Action for Neighbourhood Change

United Way (Toronto) is a Canadian NGO helping inner-city neighbour-hoods, social networks and resident associations to create meaningful partnerships in setting local priorities. United Way has made claims of significant outcomes as a result of its community-based approach,, including a fall in crime of 19 per cent in the neighbourhoods included in the programme. The programme works with people from diverse backgrounds and helps them to build the capacity, skills, knowledge and confidence they need to improve their lives. Action for Neighbourhood Change is the foundation of United Way's efforts to engage local residents through the 'building strong neighbourhoods' strategy. This strategy covers priority neighbourhoods, community groups and residents, helping to draw out existing knowledge and expertise. A Resident Action Plan was developed in each neighbourhood to identify local priorities and to guide community action. United Way offers grants directly to priority neighbourhoods to fund initiatives such as playgrounds, community gardens and kitchens to promote healthy living and recreational and cultural activities. Low-income neighbourhoods do lack supportive infrastructure: for example, social services such as employment counselling for newly arrived migrants. A supportive infrastructure for health promotion can be found not only in tangible resources and structures, but also through the extent of public and political awareness of health issues, and participation in action to address those issues (WHO, 1998). United Way has worked with other partners to establish 'community hubs' to locate several service agencies centrally, to provide easy access for local residents. Another important purpose of the community hub has been access to a community space where local resident groups can come together to hold meetings (United Way, 2012).

> Resource inputs into partnerships do not have to be financial, as people can also bring local knowledge and voluntary contributions such as their time and energy.

Active participation within partnerships can build cohesiveness between individuals that in turn can lead to better collective action (Lin, 2000). The purpose of a partnership is eventually to grow beyond local concerns and to take a stronger position on broader issues through the pooling of collective resources. Volunteers and lay workers have been an effective means to engage communities in partnerships in health promotion programmes through their active involvement in specific roles that can act as a bridge between civil society and health authorities.

Volunteers and lay health workers

> Lay health workers are members of the communities where they work, selected by the communities, answerable to the communities for their activities and supported by the health system, but not necessarily part of its organisation (WHO, 2007).

Volunteering can be defined as an activity that involves spending time doing something for free that aims to benefit the environment and others, including close relatives (Volunteering England, 2012). Volunteerism is an important aspect of working with communities and is an activity that can produce feelings of self-respect, skill development and socialisation. An important distinction is between the participation of individual volunteers and the voluntary and community sector, which provides an infrastructure for citizen involvement across the third sector. The 'third sector' is a term used to cover all not-for-profit organisations: voluntary, community, charity and social associations. There is a wide array of terms that can be used to describe lay roles, including community health advocates and educators, link workers, peer coaches and counsellors, community champions and popular opinion leaders. In particular, lay health workers have been an effective means to engage communities by actively involving them in organisation, peer education, peer support and leading opinion, and enabling them to act as a link between communities and health services (South et al., 2013).

For example, the Altogether Better project in the UK, launched in 2008, was a five-year regional–local programme designed to deliver innovative techniques to empower communities to improve their health and wellbeing. The programme focused on exceptional local volunteers who were identified as leaders to provide a focal point around which partnerships could later develop. Other participants were then drawn into the process, and with increased confidence and capacity they also became advocates for their own communities (Altogether Better, 2011).

> Volunteerism is possible at all levels of health promotion but requires people to think differently and to be prepared to trust one another (South, 2013).

Volunteers are sometimes trained in the areas in which they work, such as education and counselling, whilst others can serve on an as-needed basis, such as outreach, culturally sensitive care, home visiting, helping with transportation, and helping in community kitchens and food banks. The Cardiovascular Health Awareness Programme (CHAP) in Ontario, Canada, for example, recruits local volunteers to help carry out health checks such as measuring blood pressure. People at risk can then be referred to their doctor, helping other health professionals who would normally have to undertake this type of routine work (South et al., 2013).

Volunteers often play a pivotal role in community interventions because they provide a valuable network of local contacts and support (Winfield, 2013). Many community-based organisations depend on the efforts of hard-working volunteers who, behind the scenes, strive tirelessly doing day-to-day and often mundane activities. These volunteers receive no or low pay and can lose their motivation or become burnt out from constant struggle and slow progress. One of the most critical problems for volunteerism is the high rate of attrition, which can lead to a lack of continuity in the relationship between the programme and the community, and increases costs and time in selecting and training volunteers. Volunteers can become dissatisfied with not receiving any incentives for the services that they provide, and if this situation continues it can have a negative effect on the programme (Bhattacharya et al., 2001). Good leadership, communication and self-reflection are therefore key aspects in helping to maintain voluntary action (Frusciante, 2007).

Various incentives for volunteer retention to motivate involvement and to sustain performance have been field-tested. An international review (Bhattacharya et al., 2001) of community health workers found that successful projects had multiple incentives over time to provide better job satisfaction among the individual members. Incentives do not have to be monetary but could be in-kind such as clothing or an appreciation of their role through greater professional support.

The international review concluded that the sustainability of voluntary inputs into health programmes depends on several key factors:

- Volunteers should maintain a relationship with the community but remain accountable to them for their activities.
- The programme should plan for a high turnover of volunteers: for example, by having shorter but more regular training.
- Volunteers should continue to be made to feel valued by the health system and to collaborate with other health professionals: for example, in outreach activities.
- The spirit of volunteerism should be maintained for as long as possible, and when incentives are introduced these should be multiple and matched to duties and responsibilities.
- The volunteers should be provided with regular monitoring of their duties, and feedback (Bhattacharya et al., 2001).

The social ties that volunteerism can provide are a key determinant of health (South, 2013). However, high attrition rates and the need for regular intensive training, multiple incentives and the regular monitoring of duties mean that volunteerism is not always a cost-effective option for health promotion programmes.

Networks play an important role in supporting social relationships, including volunteerism, through a strong sense of identity and solidarity, and offer people the opportunity to access complementary resources and expertise.

Strengthening networks

A network is a structure of relationships linking people and helping to map the social connections that individuals have to one another (Pescosolido, 1991). However, networks can also affect what people do, how they feel, and what happens to them, including in regard to their health and wellbeing (Wright, 1997). A health network, for example, is a structure of relationships, both personal and professional, through which individuals maintain and receive emotional support, resources, services and information for the improvement of their health and wellbeing (Walker et al., 1977).

> In a fundamental way, our health is a reflection of the quality of our relationships with one another, which can offer people the opportunity to strengthen their health.

Health networks

Health networks can be an indication of related health behaviour: for example, the biological and behavioural traits associated with obesity appear to be spread through social ties. People who experience the weight gain of others in their social networks may then more readily accept weight gain in themselves. Moreover, social distance is more important than geographic distance within networks and there is an important role for a process involving the induction and person-to-person spread of obesity. Peer support interventions that allow for a modification of people's social networks are therefore more successful than those that do not. However, social networks can also be used to spread positive health behaviours because people's perceptions of their own risk of illness may depend on the people around them (Christakis and Fowler, 2007).

Individuals invest in and use the resources embedded in social networks because they expect returns of some sort. One cohort study in California, for example, found that survival rates from heart attack improved with an increasing level of social support. People who were socially isolated had three times the age-adjusted mortality rate than those who participated in social networks (Berkman, 1986). Individual involvement in a network can also have benefits to personal health in other ways, because networks provide sources of information about health from other members. They provide a source of emotional, practical and even financial support in times of difficultly from others in the network and an opportunity to apply pressure, through collective action (Hubley and Copeman, 2008).

Patient networks

Networks for patients can be supported by, for example, a health service agency, or may be independent and be formed by its members for the benefit of its members, both patients and health professionals. The Patients Association (UK) is a network formed around common patient issues for better information and support. The most frequent complaints received by the Patients Association are regarding poor communication, toileting, pain relief, nutrition and hydration. The Association addresses the shared concerns of its members, including the duty to refer, so that patients are able to trust their doctors to make sure they are getting access to the best treatment. Access to information is the best way to make sure this is happening, and patient support groups are ideally placed to provide this service. Doctors cannot be experts in all fields and so it is important for them to be able to direct patients to other organisations which have the expertise. Doctors can then actively support patients in finding other networks that could help them with managing their condition (Patients Association, 2011).

Building community capacity

Community capacity-building is the increase in people's abilities to define, assess, analyse and act on health (or any other) concerns of importance that they have (Labonte and Laverack, 2001).

Interest in capacity-building as a strategy for sustainable skills and resources in various health promotion settings has developed because of the requirement to prolong programme gains (Gibbon et al., 2002). In health promotion the task is not to create a new programme; rather, the task is to examine how its practice can support the development of capacity-building. Capacity-building becomes the process by which the end result of increasing programme sustainability can be achieved through increasing the knowledge, skills and competencies of programme partners.

Whilst there is clarity in regard to the definition of community capacity there is less in regard to how to make this concept operational in a programme context. In recent years, however, this concept has been 'unpacked' into the organisational areas of influence that significantly contribute to its development. The nine 'capacity domains', for example, represent those aspects of the process of community capacity that allow people to better organise and mobilise themselves towards gaining greater control over their lives. Capacities in each of the domains are indicative of a robust and capable community, one that has strong organisational and social abilities. The nine capacity domains are:

1 Improve stakeholder participation.
2 Develop local leadership.
3 Build organisational structures.
4 Increase problem assessment capacities.
5 Enhance stakeholder ability to ask 'why?
6 Improve resource mobilisation.
7 Strengthen links to other organisations and people.
8 Create an equitable relationship with outside agents.
9 Increase stakeholder control over programme management (Laverack, 2007).

A successful participatory approach to building community capacity using the nine domains has enabled people to better organise themselves, to strategically plan for actions to resolve their concerns and to evaluate the outcomes, as follows:

- A period of observation and discussion is important firstly to adapt the approach to the social and cultural requirements of the participants. For example, the use of a working definition of community capacity-building can provide all participants with a more mutual understanding of the concept in which they are involved and towards which they are expected to contribute.
- Measurement is in itself insufficient to build capacity and so this information must also be transformed into actions. This is achieved through strategic planning for positive changes in the nine domains to achieve improvements at an individual and a community level based on:
  - identifying specific activities;
  - sequencing activities into the correct order to make an improvement;
  - setting a realistic time frame including any targets; and
  - assigning individual responsibilities to complete each activity within the programme time frame.
- The resources that are necessary and available to improve the present situation are assessed.

Community capacity and heart health

Here I use a hypothetical case study to show how a community heart health programme might use each of the nine domains to build capacity.

Participation: Urging people to attend classroom-style education sessions is less likely to attract participation than organising events based around community members' interests: for example, outdoor picnics and neighbourhood tours.

Leadership: The programme used local volunteers with good networks, and good cooking, organising and child care skills, to plan community activities. They later became local leaders for a broader health promotion project aimed at a variety of issues, including housing, the environment and employment.

Organisational structures: The programme realised that the locality lacked strong community structures, and used heart health, the picnics and other initial activities to lay the framework for a new organisation. It may not always be necessary to create a new organisation, but if there are no organisations sufficiently representative of community members a new one could be developed.

Problem assessment: Health promoters helped to engage community members in problem assessment, one that incorporated both capacity-building neighbourhood needs.

Asking why: Most people are aware of heart health behaviour risks. Rather than an 'education and awareness' approach, the programme organised different educational events. These primarily consisted of working with residents in small groups to identify why some people had poorer health habits and others did not, why some people had unhealthier living conditions and others did not, and what local, state and national actions (from community members, from legislators and public policy) might remedy the unhealthy circumstances.

Resource mobilisation: Health promoters worked with the new organisation to attract resources including for issues that fell outside the funders' ideas of what were legitimate activities in relation to cardiovascular disease.

Links to others: The programme linked the new organisations to others undertaking similarly broad-based, local organising, including brokering ties with politicians and policymakers.

Outside agents: Health promoters maintained critical self-reflection on their own roles: Were they imposing? Facilitating? Empowering? This ongoing reflexive approach (see chapter 4) was evaluated periodically through assessments with community members.

Programme management: Over time, and as additional resources were obtained, the new organisation took on more direct control over programme activities (Laverack, 2004).

Visual representation of community capacity

The evaluation of community capacity has used qualitative information to provide, for example, transcribed interviews, which were difficult and time consuming to interpret. The lessons learnt from these experiences have provided the basis for new approaches that can enable people to visually represent the capacity-building process as a graphic image in a format that anyone can understand.

The purpose of visual representation is to provide a means by which to share the interpretation of the evaluation with all partners. The information can be compared over a specific time frame and between the different components of a programme. Visual representations that are culturally sensitive and are easy to reproduce can therefore be used as an appropriate tool to interpret and share qualitative information.

> The visual representation of complex concepts is an attractive option because it can show results in a way that can be easily understood by all participants.

The spider web configuration is specifically designed to be used with the 'domains approach' for building community capacity, discussed above. It can be easily constructed by using any spreadsheet package that allows quantitative values to be graphically displayed. The visual representation provides a 'snapshot' of the strengths and weaknesses of each domain and this information can be used to compare progress within a community and between communities in the same programme. Graphing differences over time allows conclusions to be drawn about the effectiveness of building community capacity in a programme context. A textual analysis should always accompany the visual representation to explain why some domains are strong and others are not (Laverack, 2007).

Figure 8.1 provides the example of a completed spider-web configuration and shows that all the 'domains' were weak at the time of making the measurement with the exception of 'resource mobilisation'. This community had previous experiences of raising funds and had therefore rated this domain higher. In particular, the domain 'programme management' was given a weak rating by the community because it was a new intervention, and a good working relationship between the community and the managers had not yet been established. Subsequent measurements can be carried out and then further plotted onto the same spider-web configuration. Over the lifetime of the programme a visual representation of community capacity, as it increases or decreases, can be plotted.

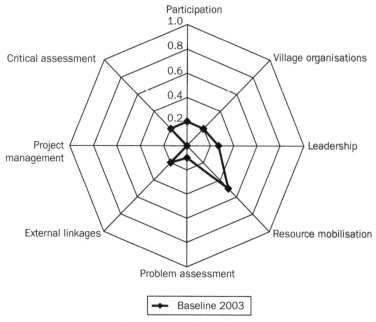

Figure 8.1 Baseline spider graph for community capacity

Key points of the chapter

- A community will occupy a spatial dimension – that is, a place or locale – and a non-spatial dimension that involves relationships between people.
- Active participation within partnerships can build the trust between individuals that in turn can lead to collective action.
- Resource inputs do not have to be financial as people can bring an intimate local knowledge and voluntary contributions such as their time and energy.
- Volunteerism is possible at all levels of health promotion, but requires people to think differently and to be prepared to trust one another.
- Capacity-building promotes programme sustainability through increasing the knowledge, skills and competencies of its partners.
- The visual representation of complex concepts is an attractive option because it can show results in a way that can be easily understood by all participants.

9 Understanding and influencing policy

Healthy public policy

Healthy public policy covers a range of activities that cut across different sectors including housing, transport and employment, and engages with a wide range of groups including consumers, government services, non-governmental organisations, pressure groups and the commercial sector (Baum, 2008).

Healthy public policy can overlap with social policy as it includes aspects of the economy, society and politics, social security and the promotion of health and education (Dixey et al., 2013). Health policy differs from healthy public policy because it is specifically concerned with the financing and operation of sickness care services and ways to address them (Brown, 1992).

It can be difficult to define the causal links between a policy intervention and an improvement in health because this is related to the social, economic and political determinants of people's lives. Policy can actually create disparities between different groups, even within the same community, and therefore developing policy solutions should involve the communities that they are designed to benefit. However, the people who control the political process (political parties and other governmental stakeholders at the national, municipal, regional and local levels) may or may not involve those who are influenced by a policy outcome. The policy process can instead be used as a means to exert control over people, resources and decision-making (Labonte and Laverack, 2008).

> Influencing policy is possible because, far from being predictable, policy is reliant on the ability of different stakeholders to negotiate a compromise in its development.

Understanding the policy process

Policy is about taking decisions, setting goals and stating ways to address them through, for example, health projects, legislation, guidelines and codes of practice. Policy development is complex and is usually made up of a combination of decisions, agendas and actions rather than just one decision, and may extend over a long period of time (Brown, 1992). Policy can change over time and is influenced by many factors, including other policy decisions and stakeholders at different levels involved in the policy formulating process. Because of the range of issues that healthy public policy addresses – for example, drinking alcohol, smoking and reducing poverty – its formulation and development is the target for pressure groups, advocacy groups and social movements, and is intrinsically a political activity (Draper, 1991). However, this can also provide the opportunity for health promoters and their partners to influence the policy process and to engage in political actions.

Policy formulation frameworks

Several useful frameworks have been developed to conceptualise how people can act to change the process of policy development (Lindquist, 2001). They primarily reflect processes in a democratic political system and within two broad paradigms: rationalist and political (Neilson, 2001).

The rationalist paradigm originates from classical economic theory, which presumes that actors have full information and are then able to establish priorities to achieve a desired and largely uncontested goal. It is driven by the production and consideration of different forms of evidence such as public health research, as well as the input from experts as a valued part of the process. The political paradigm generates policy models derived from comparative politics and international relations. These theories stress the importance of agenda setting, policy networks, policy narratives and the policy transfer in shaping final decisions. Policy decisions, in turn, are made on the basis of bargaining and negotiation between the many different stakeholders, who employ a range of approaches to have an influence on each stage of the policy process.

From the perspective of policymakers, the most effective approach combines elements from both the rational and the political paradigms. For example, the introduction of policy to ban smoking in public places was initially based on strong epidemiological evidence regarding second-hand smoke. However, the best strategy to reduce death and illness from second-hand smoke would be a total ban on smoking, including in homes. Obviously such a policy would be very difficult to regulate as well as creating opposition from civil libertarian groups. The policy decision was therefore a compromise based on the available evidence and on opposing interests to reach an achievable goal rather than an optimal goal (Neilson, 2001).

Policy development is often a compromise based on the available evidence and on opposing interests to reach an achievable, realistic goal rather than an optimal goal.

Influencing the policy process

Government action on policy can be seen as a democratic enterprise that, in theory, reflects the needs of a significant proportion of the public. The 'multiple streams model' attempts to explain agenda change: how and why some issues move onto and up the decision agenda of political parties, whilst others do not. In the 'multiple streams model' the government is viewed as an arena through which three streams of separate, simultaneous activity occur:

1 The problem stream consists of those conditions which policymakers have chosen to interpret as problems.
2 The policy stream consists of the various 'solutions' developed by specialists.
3 The politics stream consists of developments involving macropolitical conditions: the public mood, interest group politics, and turnover in the administrative and legislative stakeholders (Cohen-Vogel and McLendon, 2009).

The three streams of problems, policies and politics flow through the governmental system largely independently of one another and each according to its own set of dynamics. As a result, change within one stream may occur independently of change in the other two streams. An issue gains traction on the policy agenda only when stream convergence occurs, when a window of opportunity opens, allowing policy activists a chance to push attention towards their agenda. The extent to which public action can redefine policy concerns therefore has to wait for a development in the political stream so that activists can use this to their advantage (Cohen-Vogel and McLendon, 2009).

Six steps to influence the policy process

For those aiming to influence the policy-making process, each stage in its development offers opportunities for change. This has been defined as six steps by which outside groups can influence the policy process:

1 identify issues;
2 analyse policy;

3   undertake consultation;
4   move towards decisions;
5   implement; and
6   evaluate (Edwards et al., 2001).

1. Identify issues

Initially the health problem has to be defined and articulated before a decision can be made as to whether to include it on the policy agenda. Government policy agendas are often crowded and so issues that are to be selected are in competition with one another. It is useful if those people proposing the problem can demonstrate that it is an undesirable situation and one that is getting worse. In particular, they need to show that some public harm will result unless action is taken and that this harm can be expressed in terms of social, economic or health outcomes. For example, policy actions on smoking are more likely to be considered when the longer-term social and economic effects, such as increased health expenditure and loss in productivity, can be shown. Another example is the threat of litigation for economic costs, a strategy frequently used in the USA, which has been effective to change the production, marketing and retail practices of food companies involved in the processed and fast-food industry in regard to obesity-related damages (Labonte and Laverack, 2008).

The responsibility to place a policy issue on the government agenda usually rests with the appropriate minister, who has to ensure that there is a broad enough understanding and acceptance of the issue that it has a good chance of moving forward in the policy cycle. This provides an opportunity to influence the policy cycle through actions such as lobbying (see chapter 3): for example, by sending a letter, email or text message, or by signing a petition directed at the minister. It is also an opportunity to influence the policy cycle through actions such as taking part in peaceful demonstrations. The media can play a significant role and people can engage in a publicity campaign to try to influence the decisions made by the minister in selecting the policy agenda, for example; an issue that is obviously popular with the public may have a better chance of being placed on the policy agenda.

Having media coverage of a policy issue does not guarantee it will receive political attention, but a lack of media coverage will guarantee it gets no political attention.

Pressure groups can challenge the government for putting forward a particular policy agenda, but the success of one group's argument over another group's counter-argument is largely based on who has access to the most resources that enable them to put forward a more convincing campaign.

2. Analyse policy

Policy analysis is mostly undertaken internally and in confidence, a process in which outside influence is difficult. The steps of the policy analysis are essentially subject to internal politics but also to the politics of the state and the apparatus of administration and management. Policy analysis commonly involves three elements:

1 collecting the relevant data;
2 clarifying the objectives and resolving the key questions that have been raised; and
3 identifying the proposals that will form the basis of the policy reform.

An important factor is the level of investment made at this stage to ensure a thorough analysis of the issues and to provide sufficient clarity so that decisions can be quickly made to devise solutions to problems. But even when a policy solution exists it may have to wait for a favourable political climate. The scientific evidence against the causal link of passive smoking and ill health, for example, had existed for some time before it became a policy priority, motivated from a position of moral and personal rights. This is when the window of opportunity presented itself to act to introduce policy on passive smoking with the support of the public (Berridge, 2007).

> Researchers can play an important but limited role in helping to identify and provide the evidence necessary to resolve issues arising during the policy analysis.

A few researchers are able to engage with policy analysis directly through advisory boards, ministerial briefings and research partnerships with government. Researchers try to facilitate the use of their work by providing scientifically rigorous evidence; however, the academic language and lengthy publication timescales often miss the rapidly shifting arena of policy development. Researchers can offer formal advice, making themselves available to policymakers for consultation and providing expedited reports and reviews. On the other hand, policymakers interpret research-informed advice for inspiration and for pragmatic operational reasons. They are savvy, somewhat cynical operators in a political arena who use researchers for their own ends.

This does depend on the role and position of the researcher, the current stage of policy development in which they are engaged, the level of contention about the policy and the researchers' credibility. For example, high-profile researchers with a vision of their field and rhetorical skills are used to persuade ministers, stakeholders and the public during policy agenda setting and formation. Researchers with a narrower expertise, such as specialists in clinical trials, are used to advise on intervention design and evaluation once overall policy directions have been agreed (Haynes et al., 2011).

In reality, policy development is mostly undertaken internally, and in confidence, and the level of public involvement and researcher consultation is limited.

3. Undertake consultation

Consultation can be formal or informal and may occur at any stage of the policy process. Consultation is often facilitated by the issue of a discussion paper which outlines the policy intentions and allows feedback from individuals and pressure groups. People may be formally asked for a response to the discussion paper or it may be placed in the public arena to stimulate an open debate on the issues. The purpose is that the consultation stage will lead to a refinement of the policy and a wider public acceptance of its intentions.

It is at this stage that there is an opportunity for engagement in the policy process. The New Zealand Prostitutes Collective (NZPC), for example, was able to bring about a change in legislation through the Prostitution Reform Act 2003. This was largely achieved through their collective action and, critically, because of their internal access to government advisory committees on HIV/AIDS. A major factor leading to the NZPC having a greater influence was the desire of public health authorities to communicate with the sex industry to address the spread of HIV. This provided the impetus for the offer of support and collaboration with government advisory committees and gave the NZPC a privileged position that allowed it to shift the agenda to include the rights, occupational health and safety of sex workers (Laverack and Whipple, 2010).

The evidence on influencing policy suggests that internal access to policy shops and advisory committees can be an effective strategy.

The purpose at this stage is to ensure that the people involved in making the decisions are aware of public opinion for or against the issue, and consultation is especially important when policy choices are strongly contested. Whilst the move to community consultation by governments is a potentially positive step it is not always clear whose interests are being served most. Participation may become a way of demonstrating a democratic process that is actually devoid of critical reflection on how it might be empowering for the communities affected. In the end, bureaucrats become more empowered because they can claim to have consulted with the community, and therefore their conclusions have more politically correct weight. If these conclusions truly do benefit community groups, this is not necessarily a bad outcome. But that may not always be the case, and unless practitioners are clear on the reasons why they are consulting with communities they risk engaging them in discussions of no real importance.

4. Move towards decisions

Following analysis, debate and refinement of the policy a proposal will be put forward for approval by the government or relevant agency. In spite of the earlier analysis and consultation, the final decision will still have to consider issues of economy, efficiency and equity. A compromise may have to be reached: for example, one in which the policy is phased in over a period of time to allow sufficient funds to be made available. Alternatively, the policy reforms may be introduced as a package alongside other measures, assistance and benefits. The purpose is to publicly introduce the policy reform with a minimum of opposition and criticism.

At this stage of the policy process, if people are opposed to the decisions they can continue to use a range of direct and indirect actions such as the threat of collectively withdrawing their votes for those making the decision, engaging in an aggressive publicity campaign or instigating legal action against those making the policy decision. The purpose of these actions is to try to force those making the policy decision to agree upon a compromise in favour of the opinions of those against it.

5. Implement

Once the decisions have been made and approved the policy enters a period of implementation towards the desired outcomes although this invariably entails some modification. The evidence shows a number of causes for a failure at the implementation stage including ambiguity in the policy itself, conflict with other policies, having a low political priority or engendering conflict with significant stakeholders (Edwards et al., 2001).

Policies can actually be reformulated at the implementation stage, and this provides the opportunity to interfere with and possibly stall the process of implementation. The best chance of success at this stage is the effect of bad publicity that can be harnessed against the policy reform. To do this, innovative communication technology (see chapter 3) such as texting e-petitions can be used as a low-cost but effective option. This is possible because at this stage decision-makers often lose interest in the policy process and insufficient resources are given to promote the reforms.

6. Evaluate

Evaluation is an essential part of the process of formulation and implementation and allows information to be continually fed back to adapt, change or even cancel policy. The evaluation of the policy can lead to incremental revisions if reforms are not being met efficiently: for example, if the purpose of the reform was to increase equity in child support but this was later shown not to have happened, the policy may be changed and re-implemented. The evaluation can be influenced by a broader political agenda which may also have changed since the original policy decision was made. It may then be more difficult to justify a continuation of the policy if, for example, it now has a lower priority in the political agenda. Policy evaluation gives further hope to those who, if their actions and tactics to influence it have been unsuccessful, can use the revision process as a means to reintroduce changes or to stop the reforms.

Health impact assessment is a means of assessing the health impacts of policies by using quantitative, qualitative and participatory techniques. For example, transport is a major factor in traffic injuries, air pollution and noise. Healthy transport policy can help reduce these risks, as well as promoting physical activity such as walking and cycling (Taylor et al., 2003).

> The success of influencing the policy process is increased when it is technically simple and necessitates only marginal changes in any existing policy.

The likelihood of success of influencing the policy process is further increased when it is delivered by one agency, has clear objectives, has a short duration (Walt, 1994) and addresses medically defined problems rather than those residing in the complex social determinants of health.

The influence of civil society organisations

Health promoters play an integral part in the implementation of policy through the programmes they deliver aimed at improving health. The practitioner can also use their knowledge, resources and expertise to work with civil society groups to help them gain more control over the policy process. Because of the range of issues that healthy public policy addresses, for example – drinking alcohol and smoking – its formulation is also the target for pressure groups, social movements and activists, and is intrinsically a political activity (Draper, 1991). The competing interests involved in many decisions around healthy public policy mean that its implementation will also often result in challenging the authority of some stakeholders who have a great deal of influence and who wish to protect the interests of their shareholders, employees and members. Civil society organisations therefore have to use a variety of tactics to achieve their goals and to have more political influence.

Pressure groups

> The aim of pressure groups is to change the opinions and attitudes of society and to influence the policy-making process (Young and Everritt, 2004).

Pressure groups are commonly formed on the basis of the interests of their members including professional and community-based organisations, for a particular cause. There is an important distinction to be made between pressure groups that are supported by an outside agent such as a health service employer, and those that are independent and are formed by its members, for the benefit of its members.

Health consumer groups

Health consumer groups are voluntary organisations that promote and represent the interests of the users or carers of health services, usually formed at a national level by its members, for the benefit of its members (Allsop et al., 2004). These groups cover a range of health conditions including heart disease, mental health, and maternal and child health. Health consumer groups are mostly charitable organisations and are focused on one particular policy issue, choosing to use tactics such as sharing information, providing support services for their members and using online resources.

A practical example is the action of women in the UK who established local pressure groups to organise and mobilise themselves to try to bring about a change in the decision made by the National Health Service trusts to refuse to fund the drug Herceptin® for use in the early stages of breast cancer, until it was licensed. They organised actions such as local demonstrations outside hospitals, petitions, sit-in protests and letters and emails to their Members of Parliament. They established a website to support other women and embarked on an aggressive publicity campaign against the government. Eventually, the success of a court case ensured that Herceptin® was approved for use on the National Health Service. This was largely because of the determined action of the pressure group at the national level, which in turn had a wider influence on the distribution of Herceptin® to others (Boseley, 2006).

It should be noted that pressure groups can simply become actors in a process that actually enhances the legitimacy of government policy or corporate interests as these pursue their own agenda. This is because pressure groups are usually short-term and often have little influence and few resources. However, their chances of success are enhanced if they are able to form some kind of an alliance or partnership with others that share their concerns to create a broader health social movement.

Health social movements

Health social movements challenge state, institutional and other forms of authority to give the public more of a voice in policy development (Brown and Zavestoski, 2004).

Health social movements are an important point of social interaction concerning the rights of people to access services and to address inequalities based on, for example, race, class, gender and sexuality. What makes a movement different from other forms of social mobilisation, such as pressure and advocacy groups, is an ability to go beyond the influence of its participant and resource base. A social movement is able to maintain an ideology irrespective of membership, function and organisational structure. To do this, a movement must have 'deep social roots' and strong social networks (Laverack, 2013b).

Health social movements overlap in their purpose and tactics but can be broadly categorised into three types:

1 Health access movements seek equitable access to healthcare services: for example, through national healthcare reforms and an extension of health insurance to non-insured sectors of the population.
2 Embodied health movements are concerned with people who want to address personal experiences of disease, illness and disability through a challenge of the scientific evidence by medical recognition of their ideas or their own research. They can include people

directly affected by a condition or those who feel they are an at-risk group: for example, the HIV/AIDS movement.

3 Constituency-based health movements concern health inequalities when the evidence shows an oversight or disproportionate outcome: for example, the human rights movement (Brown and Zavestoski, 2004).

The negative publicity received about, for example, experimentation with contraceptives, radiation and immunisation, has created a heightened level of distrust by the public and has led to people challenging government policy. People have discovered that collectively, through for example health social movements, they can apply significant pressure to influence the policy that affects their lives and health (Brown and Zavestoski, 2004).

> Social movements are important to health promotion because they provide the opportunity for people to have greater influence through a broad participant and resource base.

The environmental breast cancer movement

The environmental breast cancer movement in the USA is an example of the efforts of women who were concerned with both inequitable access to healthcare services and human rights. This health social movement was created in the 1970s in the San Francisco Bay area by those at risk from or affected by breast cancer. The health social movement pressed for expanded clinical trials, compassionate access to new drugs and greater government funding, using tactics such as engaging in legal action and creative media campaigns to influence the policy process (Brown and Zavestoski, 2004). Twenty years later a new regime of breast cancer had emerged, influenced by the efforts of the environmental breast cancer movement. Women had access to user-friendly cancer centres, patient education and support groups, a choice of medical alternatives and a role as part of the healthcare team that delivered the cancer treatment. Essentially, breast cancer became politicised and was reframed as a human rights issue and an environmental disease (Klawiter, 2004).

Health activism

> Health activism involves a challenge to the existing order whenever it is perceived to influence people's health negatively or has led to an injustice or an inequity (Plows, 2007).

Activism is action on behalf of a cause: action that goes beyond what is routine and conventional in society (Martin, 2007), and therefore is relative to other actions used by individuals, groups and organisations. Activism has an explicit purpose to help to empower others, and this is embodied in actions that are typically energetic, passionate, innovative and committed. Historically, activism has played a major role in protecting workers from exploitation, protecting the environment, promoting equality for women and opposing racism (Laverack, 2013b).

Indirect and direct actions

The types of actions that activist organisations engage in can be broadly sub-divided into two categories: indirect and direct.

1 Indirect actions are non-violent and conventional and often require a minimum of effort, although collectively they can have a dramatic effect. Indirect actions include voting, signing a petition, taking part in a 'virtual (online) sit-in' and sending a letter or email to protest about your cause.
2 Direct actions can become progressively more 'unconventional', ranging from peaceful protests to inflicting intentional physical damage on persons and property.

For most activists their focus is on short-term, reactive, direct tactics as their primary, and often only, means of action, aiming to have a real-time and immediate effect.

Direct actions can be further sub-divided into non-violent and violent actions.

Non-violent direct actions include protests, picketing, vigils, marches, rent strikes, consumer boycotts, publicity campaigns and taking legal action. The purpose of these tactics is to add to the level of influence that an individual, group or organisation has by harnessing additional assets.

Consumer boycotts, for example, are a form of non-violent direct action focused on the long-term change of buying habits and are usually part of a larger strategy aiming for the reform of consumer markets, or government commitment to the moral purchasing of products. Consumer boycotting was a tactic of activists in the 1960s and 1970s to try to punish corporations. By the 1990s, however, the trend was more towards developing standards and accrediting retail products that would be rewarded by consumers. Concerns have been raised that boycotting products may force the people involved in the labour of manufacture to turn to more dangerous sources of income. UNICEF, for example, has estimated that 50,000 children were dismissed from their garment industry jobs in Bangladesh following the introduction of the Child Labour Deterrence Act in the USA in the 1990s. Many children then resorted to jobs such as stone-crushing, street hustling and prostitution, jobs that are more hazardous and exploitative than garment production. The study suggests that some product boycotts can have long-term negative consequences that actually harm rather than help children employed in low-income jobs (UNICEF, 2001).

Direct violent actions include physical tactics used against people or property, placing oneself in a position of manufactured vulnerability to prevent action or taking part in a civil disobedience. Direct action can be symbolic and challenging, sending a message to the general public, and/or to the owners, shareholders and employees of a specific company, and/or to policymakers, about specific grievances.

The range of tactics used by activists extends from conventional, peaceful tactics to increasingly unconventional and more violent actions. If the use of conventional tactics by an organisation is not successful then it may choose to use more radical tactics as a part of its long-term strategy. This is a dynamic process because organisations also use a variety of tactics, culturally informed and to some extent shaped by local laws. The tactics also continue to evolve along with political opportunity and developments in technology including the use of innovative communication technologies to carry out online tactics.

Key points of the chapter

- Influencing policy is possible because the policy process is reliant on the ability of the different stakeholders to negotiate a compromise in its development.
- Policy is often a compromise based on the available evidence and on opposing interests to reach an achievable, realistic goal rather than an optimal goal.
- Policy development is mostly undertaken internally, and in confidence, and the level of public involvement and researcher consultation is limited.
- Direct actions through pressure groups, social movements and activism can be an effective way to influence the policy development process.

The evaluation of health promotion

Evaluation is concerned with the assessment of how actions have achieved a specific outcome or how far a change has taken place in the intended target group as a result of the health promotion programme (Hubley and Copeman, 2013).

What is evaluation?

The evaluation of health promotion is an evolving field aiming to provide more evidence of what really works. This is made more difficult because of the wide range of approaches, models and theories that are used in health promotion, and the financial, time and capacity constraints that health promoters face in practice.

Health promotion programmes are delivered to promote or maintain the health and wellbeing of an individual, group or community. Whilst there is no real agreement about the overall purpose of a programme evaluation it should address the overall goals and provide information about the process, outcomes, impact, operation, progress and achievements. The evaluation helps to understand what happens during the programme period (and beyond), both positively and negatively, to learn from it and then to draw evidence-based conclusions.

Health promoters are increasingly being asked to provide evidence that their practice is effective even though the theories and approaches that they use are often considered to be untested (Raphael, 2000).

Top-down and bottom-up styles of evaluation

Health promotion evaluation has traditionally used predetermined indicators towards which the beneficiaries of the programme do not usually contribute. The role of the health promoter has been as an 'expert', one who judges merit or worth. The evaluation has been used as an instrument of control through performance measurement, the achievement of targets and by providing feedback about the operational elements of the implementation. This is a top-down style of evaluation that can be disempowering to all stakeholders of the programme.

A bottom-up style of evaluation places the focus on involving all the partners through participatory methods and moves practice away from conventional 'expert'-driven approaches. This means a fundamental shift between the practitioners and the beneficiaries of the programme, one where control over decisions about the evaluation are more equitably distributed. The evaluation helps to empower the beneficiaries by actively involving them in the process of evaluation and skills development to subsequently provide the means to improve the programme further (Laverack, 2007).

> The evaluation of health promotion is seldom perfect, often messy, 'quick and dirty' or even omitted. This can be avoided by allowing sufficient resources for an evaluation and by following a few simple steps during the programme planning.

Six simple steps for programme evaluation

Evaluation is typically carried out during the programme delivery or after it has been completed and this can be strengthened by following, as closely as possible within the constraints of the implementation, six simple steps during planning:

1 Set SMART (Specific, Measurable, Achievable, Realistic and Time-scaled) objectives at the beginning of the programme.
2 Carry out a baseline study to be able to demonstrate any changes as a result of the programme activities.
3 Address process, outcome and impact, and look for achievements as well as programme failures in the design of the evaluation.
4 If possible, identify controls (identical or similar situations) to be able to show change as a result of the programme activities.
5 Involve all partners in the evaluation.
6 Plan to record programme benefits that might otherwise be missed by the evaluation: for example, 'spin-offs' such as an increase in community cohesion (Hubley and Copeman, 2013).

Two paradigms of evaluation

When applying a research approach to the evaluation it is first helpful to consider the use of an appropriate paradigm. A paradigm can be defined as a world view that is composed of multiple belief

categories, principal among them being their ontological, epistemological and methodological assumptions (Guba, 1990). Ontological
assumptions are about the way in which the world is, the nature of
reality. Epistemological assumptions are about what we can know
about that reality. Methodological assumptions are about how we
come to know that reality and the strategies we employ in order to
discover the way in which the world functions. Two paradigms that
are the most relevant to the evaluation of health promotion are positivist and constructivist.

The positivist paradigm

The conventional health promotion paradigm is typified as positivist.
Its ontology consists of a belief in a single reality, independent of any
observer, and a belief that universal truths, independent of time and
place, exist and can be discovered. Its epistemology consists of a belief
that the evaluator can and should investigate a phenomenon in a way
that is uncluttered by values and biases. The methodology favours
experimental designs to test hypotheses and is concerned with predic-
tion through proof or certainty and with singular measures of reality
and truth (Labonte and Robertson, 1996).

The constructivist paradigm

The constructivist paradigm provides a wider framework in which
'truth' and 'fact' are recognised for having subjective dimensions.
What emerges from this process is an agenda for negotiation based on
the issues raised between the evaluator and those involved in the evaluation. Its ontology is relativist, meaning that realities are socially
constructed. Realities are local and specific, dependent on their form
and content and on the persons who hold them. Its epistemology recognises the evaluator as part of the reality that is being evaluated, and
the findings are a creation of the inquiry process between the inquirer
and inquired. In the constructivist paradigm truth is not absolute, but
rather is understood as the best-informed and most sophisticated truth
we might construct at any given moment. The methodology uses qualitative interviewing and observation techniques that seek to know
how and what people experience within their context. Individual con-
structions are elicited, refined, compared and contrasted using, for
example, a textual analysis of the information, with the aim of gen-
erating one or more interpretations (Labonte and Robertson, 1996).
The constructivist paradigm is well suited to participatory evaluation
techniques in health promotion that purposefully involves all the programme stakeholders.

It is a constructivist paradigm that can best accommodate the methodological, epistemological and ontological assumptions of a health promotion evaluation.

Evidence-based practice

Evidence-based practice, in whatever professional context, involves not only scientific evidence but the judgement (knowledge and experience) of the practitioner and of their programme partners (Craig and Smyth, 2002).

Practitioners are under pressure to document the changes they bring about, consistent with the programme aims and objectives. The movement to develop an 'evidence-based practice' first began in the field of medicine but quickly spread to other parts of the health sector, including health promotion. The movement addresses the integration of systematically derived knowledge with the practitioner's own experience and their interpretation of the needs of the people with whom they work.

Best practice refers to the knowledge, tools and strategies which have been evaluated and are accepted as being effective. The impetus to broaden the health promotion agenda has been reinforced by concerns about the variable effectiveness of past health promotion initiatives and the increased understanding of growing inequalities in health. The development of an evidence-based practice must therefore be examined in the light of the growing need for effective interventions that address the determinants of health, in addition to individuals' behavioural risk factors (Rychetnik and Wise, 2004).

Much of what counts as evidence is a contested issue because it is not always possible to measure the important aspects of health promotion work.

The challenges of an evidence-based practice include the poor availability of information from evaluation findings and from expert knowledge. Evidence-based knowledge is not comprehensive and there are gaps in the research about the effectiveness of what health promoters do in their daily work. Evidence-based practice relies on the findings of research to be transferable into the work setting. This is not necessarily the case, as academics often do not understand the work context; neither are practitioners always skilled enough to appraise what works and what does not work for their professional context from academic publications.

Evaluating health promotion

At a pragmatic level the evaluation of health promotion should focus on the use of an evidence-based approach and the need to use realistic processes and outcomes in a programme context. However, it can be difficult to trace the pathways that link particular health promotion actions to specific long-term health or social outcomes such as a reduction in poor health or disability. This can result in a diminished value being attributed to the role of health promotion, and this is not helped by the confounding factors of isolating cause and effect in complex lifestyle situations (see table 10.1).

Table 10.1 Different types of health promotion evaluation

Sequence	Description	Measures
Formative evaluation	Is used to develop and sometimes to pre-test materials and methods as a part of programme planning, and therefore occurs prior to implementation.	Relevance, reliability and validity of specific materials and methods. For example, the piloting of leaflets and posters to raise awareness on a specific health issue.
Process evaluation	Is used to assess how the programme works once it has started and the extent to which it is being delivered effectively.	Health promotion outcomes or modifiable personal, social and environmental factors that are a means to changing the determinants of health. For example, knowledge, skills, participation and organisation.
Impact evaluation	Is used to assess its objectives or short-term progress in the implementation of the programme.	Intermediate health outcomes including in lifestyle factors such as increased physical activity or a reduction in calorie intake. Also the improved utilisation of health services or political action through, for example, patient pressure groups.

(continued)

Table 10.1 (*Continued*)

Sequence	Description	Measures
Outcome evaluation	Is used to assess whether or not the programme has achieved its aims or longer-term changes.	Long-term health and social outcomes: for example, reduced disability and avoidable mortality or changes in healthy public policy and reductions in health inequalities.

Bamberger et al. (2006) provide a simple approach that captures the essence of evaluation and places an emphasis on methodological rigour in health promotion programmes.

> As a general rule of thumb, between 5 and 10 per cent of the total programme budget should be used for the purposes of monitoring and evaluation.

- The planning and scoping of the evaluation are followed by strategies to address the budget constraints of the programme.
- The evaluation must take into account any time constraints of a new or ongoing programme and any problems for collecting data.
- The issue of political influences in the design, implementation and dissemination of the findings is an important consideration.
- Important findings can be lost and are not effectively used in improving future programmes unless properly disseminated, validated and utilised for improving health.

In practice, the evaluation must at least provide information that shows whether or not the programme activities have been implemented effectively (the process evaluation) and if it has efficiently met its stated aims (the outcome evaluation).

Process evaluation

> Process evaluation aims to understand how the programme worked, what actually happened and how people reacted to it (Nutbeam and Bauman, 2006).

To achieve its aims the programme must firstly engage with its partners, involve them in the implementation of the strategy and use relevant methods to evaluate what happened. A process evaluation is best
carried out during the delivery of the programme in a systematic way
that describes the reach of the programme, its strengths and weaknesses and why it has or has not worked in practice.

> Process evaluation is sometimes not well performed or may be omitted
> because practitioners are expected to deliver activities and services.

The process evaluation allows health promoters to be more aware
of the effectiveness of their work and the influence of what they do
on the progress of the programme. It involves the collection, collation
and analysis of qualitative and quantitative information at both the
individual and collective levels. The tools and instruments to collect
the information include surveys and questionnaires, simple counts of
attendance, a demonstration of improved knowledge and skill levels, and
reported satisfaction in the delivery of a service. The process evaluation
can also be measured by using health promotion outcomes because these
represent the most immediate results of inputs. These are modifiable personal, social and environmental factors that are a means to changing the
determinants of health: for example, knowledge, skills, social norms and
personal actions for health (Nutbeam and Bauman, 2006).

Monitoring progress

Monitoring is the systematic and routine collection of information,
often as a part of the process evaluation, and has five key purposes:

1 To learn from experiences to improve practices and activities in the
   future.
2 To have internal and external accountability of the resources used
   and the results obtained.
3 To take informed decisions on the future of the initiative.
4 To promote empowerment of beneficiaries of the initiative.
5 To assess progress and then to feed this back into the implementation of the programme to improve its delivery (Nutbeam and
   Bauman, 2006).

Monitoring is a periodically recurring task beginning in the planning
stage of a programme and allows results, processes and experiences to
be documented and used as the basis to steer decision-making. The information acquired through monitoring is often included in the evaluation to

better understand the ways in which the programme has developed over time and how this can be improved or changed.

Outcome evaluation

> Outcome evaluation aims to assess whether or not the programme has achieved its goals as well as any longer-term changes (Nutbeam and Bauman, 2006).

Outcome evaluation is often defined against a predetermined benchmark so that progress made, or not, can be measured. Setting targets requires the existence of information about the distribution of that indicator within a population. Health targets, for example, require an estimate of current and likely future trends in relation to change in the distribution of the indicator, and an understanding of the potential to change the distribution of the indicator in the population (WHO, 1998). This type of information is also provided in health profiles as a summary of health and social information for a particular population and sub-divided into regions, provinces, towns and local communities.

Outcome evaluation is measured using long-term health and social outcomes. Health outcomes are usually assessed using indicators that can be used to describe one or more measurable aspects of the health of an individual or population over the programme period. Health indicators include the measurement of illness or disease, or positive aspects of health such as quality of life, and of behaviours and actions which are related to healthy lifestyles such as physical activity. Social outcomes include indicators which measure the social and economic conditions as they relate to health and also measure changes in healthy public policy (WHO, 1998): for example, levels of disability, inequality and mental health in society.

The indicators of an outcome evaluation are often long term, complex and difficult to measure within the relatively short-term time frame of a programme. Process and outcome indicators should therefore always be used together to provide a more holistic evaluation of a health promotion programme.

Assessing change

There are at least three ways to assess change that can be attributed to health promotion programmes:

1 A randomised control trial involves measuring the impact of the programme on a specific target group and comparing this with any impact on an identical group (the control) that has not been exposed to the health promotion intervention.

2 A quasi-experimental design involves measuring the impact of the programme on a specific target group and comparing this with any impact on a similar group matched by characteristics such as age, education and income, and that has not been exposed to the health promotion intervention.

3 A before and after study has no control or comparison group and the attributing causality is ascertained by asking partners why they had changed using, for example, a self-reporting questionnaire, a focus group or one-to-one interview (Jirojwong and Liamputtong, 2009).

Assessment of change can be further verified through a triangulation of the information provided in other sources such as programme plans, practitioner logs, minutes of meetings and activity reports. Triangulation refers to the use of a variety of quantitative and qualitative methods, and a number of evaluators each with differing points of view, to evaluate the same change (Sechrest, 1997).

Evaluation that promotes participation and empowerment

Methods for evaluation use existing data, household surveys and individual questionnaires, observation techniques and in-depth interviewing. In practice, the participation of those involved is more likely to be the representation of the majority by a few: for example, through a sample of the community or elected individuals taking part in a meeting. The methodology must then contextualise the important issues, often through participatory methods, so that they are relevant to the broader population. Care must be taken to avoid the evaluation becoming empty and frustrating for those whose involvement is passive and that in effect allows those in authority to claim that all sides were considered whilst only a few benefited.

Participatory evaluation

There is a range of participatory methodologies that have been designed to actively involve people in the gathering of information. The advantages of using a participatory evaluation over conventional assessments in health promotion programmes include:

1 it is self-educative;
2 it is self-improving;

3 it enables stakeholders to monitor progress; and
4 it builds upon and improves skills (Mays and Pope, 1995).

It should be noted that a limitation of using participatory techniques is that they require skilled facilitation. Within a health promotion programme this may sometimes not be realistic to achieve because of a lack of professional competence and confidence in using participatory approaches.

Participatory rural appraisal (PRA), for example, is an approach that is used in practice as it offers a collection of methods to enable people to collect, share and analyse information that they themselves have identified as being important. However, whilst PRA can produce a large amount of information it does not always offer a means to transform this into action, a crucial stage in evaluation that promotes empowerment.

> Participatory evaluation that does not offer the means to transform information into action is only a needs assessment, rather than being an empowering experience.

In a practical sense, the participatory evaluation should be based on the shared experiences of the participants which, as far as possible, are not influenced by the methodology or have not been biased by the evaluator. However, an evaluator's presence will always influence the findings of the evaluation. Even at the most basic level, having an evaluator observing actions may affect the validity of information by stimulating modifications in behaviour or self-questioning among those participating (Mays and Pope, 1995). The participants themselves may also be a source of 'subject bias': for example, participants, knowing the importance or reward they will receive from a good result or the result desired by the evaluator, will change their behaviour or make a stronger effort during an evaluation.

Validity in participatory evaluation

Validity in using qualitative evaluation can be problematic, for at least three reasons:

1 to an extent, people are assessing their own work;
2 perceptions are prone to recall bias; and
3 the assessment may be influenced by the dynamics of the group, the evaluator or the techniques used (Nutbeam and Bauman, 2006).

Guba and Lincoln (1989) suggest the following considerations for a participatory evaluation that can be applied to help maintain rigour, validity and credibility:

- Verification of data with stakeholders: for example, to cross-check cultural interpretations.
- Triangulation using different methods and data sources.
- A clear documentation of the process from data collection to conclusions.
- Verification of interpretations by other evaluators through inter-observer agreement.
- Critical self-reflection on meanings of the findings and relevance to stakeholders.

Validity concerns can be further offset by having an emphasis on people providing reasons and examples for their assessments: for example, by providing a brief account of the history and context of the conclusions reached by the individual or group (Bell-Woodard et al., 2005).

Community stories

Community stories are a tried and tested way to involve others in an evaluation and to promote participation and empowerment. Community stories can be used to identify important needs and to help build a mutual understanding of the outcomes of the evaluation (Wood et al., 1998).

Storytelling can be initiated through group discussion and the voicing of individual and collective experience. Various techniques can be used to stimulate this process, including using photographs, or encouraging the participants to draw a picture or to create a song. People describe the stories that they create using these techniques and this in turn provides more meaning and context.

Three techniques that have been successfully used for developing community stories are:

1 'unserialised posters';
2 the 'three-pile sorting cards'; and
3 'story with a gap'.

Unserialised posters

The separate unserialised posters are prepared in advance as pictures: for example, cuttings from magazines, photographs or hand-drawn diagrams. The pictures show a variety of situations relevant to the community, such as a road traffic accident, about which the group members are asked to select four of the unserialised posters and to then develop a story using the images. The group is asked to give names to the people and places in the pictures and to give the story a beginning, a middle and an end. The group is asked to present the story to other participants, who are encouraged to ask questions about it. In particular, the facilitator should ask:

- Are these stories about events in your community?
- What issues have been raised that could be considered to be needs in your community?
- How could these be resolved?

The facilitator keeps a record of the needs that have been identified during the presentation of the story. These points are then used to generate a discussion with the group on what it has learnt and what needs it feels could be addressed by the community. The facilitator can help the community by developing a strategy to then address its concerns through identifying realistic actions and resources (Wood et al., 1998).

Three-pile sorting cards

The three-pile sorting cards are a technique that can be used to develop a story about the causes of poor health as well as other problems in the community. A set of 15 cards, each with a picture that can be interpreted as either good, bad or in-between, from a health (or any other) perspective, are distributed among the participants. Some examples in regard to a healthier lifestyle and nutrition are provided in table 10.2.

The task of the participants is to sort the 15 cards into the three categories (good, bad or in-between), to reconsider their choices and then to share their conclusions with the facilitators or with other group members. The participants are asked to select one card or more from the 'bad' category and to create a list of actions to resolve the problems using another selection of cards from the 'good' category. The participants have to decide the reasons for the 'bad' situation, who is responsible and how to address the issue: for example, through the use of a strategic plan detailing when, who and what is needed to address the issue. The participants can also identify potential partners to help them, such as a government agency, or friends and family (Srinivasan, 1993).

Table 10.2 Nutrition examples for a three-pile sorting card activity

Good	Bad	In-between
Vegetables	Sugary drinks	Weighing oneself
Physical activity	Fast food	Shopping for food
Fruit	Large portions of food	Eating a snack
Small plate portion	Watching television	Watching people play sport

The story with a gap

The story with a gap is an established approach that can be used to stimulate discussion about the needs of a community in a participatory way. Each group of community representatives is given two large pictures. One picture shows the before situation of a community problem or need: for example, anti-social behaviour in a local park. The second picture shows the after situation: for example, families in the park and children using the playground. The group is asked to develop a story which explains how this improvement has occurred. The stories that they develop will 'fill the gap' between the two pictures. The group members are asked to recount their stories and the content is discussed to identify possible pathways to find solutions. The facilitator can help with this process of discovery and learning (Srinivasan, 1993).

Key points of the chapter

- The evaluation of health promotion is an evolving field with the need to provide more evidence of what really works.
- Health promoters are increasingly being asked to provide evidence that practice is effective even though the approaches that they use are often untested.
- The evaluation of health promotion is seldom perfect, and often messy or even omitted.
- The assessment of change should be validated and verified using techniques such as a triangulation of the findings.
- Techniques such as community stories are a good way of promoting participation and empowerment in the evaluation.

PART III
Further reading

Glossary of terms

Advocacy People acting on behalf of themselves or on behalf of others to argue a position and to influence the outcome of decisions.

Alliance A relationship between two or more parties (individuals, groups, communities or organisations) to pursue a set of agreed upon goals whilst remaining independent organisations.

Asset-based community development (ABCD) A methodology that seeks to use the strengths or assets within communities as a means for more sustainable development.

Best practice The knowledge, tools and strategies which have been evaluated and are accepted as being effective.

Bottom-up An approach to help people to identify and act on their health needs in collaboration with those who have the decision-making authority.

Boycott An act of voluntarily abstaining from using, buying or dealing with a person, organisation or product as an expression of protest, usually for political reasons.

Coalition A temporary arrangement that is formed to work around one specific issue often with another organisation.

Community capacity-building The increase in community groups' abilities to define, assess, analyse and act on health (or any other) concerns of importance to their members.

Conflict resolution Methods used in facilitating the peaceful ending of conflict by individuals or group members by actively communicating information about their conflicting motives or ideologies to others and by engaging in collective negotiation.

Consumer boycott A boycott that is focused on long-term change of buying habits and usually part of a larger strategy aiming for the reform of commodity markets, or government commitment to moral purchasing of products.

Corporate social responsibility A form of self-regulation integrated into a business plan or model.

Counselling Any form of interaction where someone seeks to explore, understand or resolve a problem or a troubling personal aspect of their life.

Critical consciousness The ability to understand the causes of one's powerlessness by reflecting on the assumptions underlying our and others' ideas and actions.

Determinants of health   The determinants of health encompass the economic and social conditions that influence the health of individuals, communities and populations.

Downstream approach   The individual level in which people may be targeted for a condition or risk such as screening for early signs of breast cancer.

Empowerment   A process by which communities gain more control over the decisions and resources that influence their lives and health.

Equity   A normative judgement of what is fair.

Evaluation   Concerned with the assessment of the extent to which actions have achieved a specific outcome or that a change has taken place in the intended target group as a result of the programme.

Evidence-based practice   Involves the judgements of practitioners, programme partners and a systematic appraisal of research, theory and models.

Formative evaluation   Is used to develop and pre-test materials and methods as a part of programme planning.

Grounded citizens' jury   An approach for local involvement in health decision-making that can be used as a 'grounded' tool in which people are the agents in the development of actions directly affecting their lives.

Harm reduction   A pragmatic approach to reduce the harmful consequences of high-risk behaviours by incorporating strategies that cover safer use, managed use and abstinence.

Health activism   A challenge to the existing order whenever it is perceived to influence people's health negatively or has led to an injustice or an inequity.

Health impact assessment   A means of assessing the health impacts of policies in diverse economic sectors using quantitative, qualitative and participatory techniques.

Health in All Policies   An approach which emphasises that wellbeing is largely influenced by government sectors other than health, and which highlights the interactions between different policies.

Health inequity   Is a difference (an inequality) in health (however measured) that is significant in size and number of people affected, preventable through policy or another intervention and not an effect of freely chosen risk.

Health literacy   Focused on skills development so as to help others to make informed decisions that will allow them to exert greater control over their lives and health.

Health policy   Specifically concerned with the financing and operation of sickness care services and ways to address them through, for example, health programmes, legislation, guidelines and codes of practice.

Healthy public policy   A range of activities and decisions that cut across different sectors – for example, housing, transport and employment – and that influence quality of life, wellbeing and health.

Impact evaluation Is used to assess the objectives or short-term progress in the implementation of a programme.

Information and communication technology (ICT) The integration of telecommunications, computers, software and audio-visuals that enables users to create, access, store, transmit and manipulate information.

Lay epidemiology A term to describe the processes by which people in their everyday life understand and interpret risks, including risks to their health and wellbeing.

Lay health worker Member of the community where they work, selected by the community, answerable to the community but supported by the health system, although not necessarily part of its organisation.

Learned helplessness The condition of learning to behave in a powerless way, failing to respond even though there are opportunities to help oneself.

Learned optimism People consciously challenging any negative aspects in their lives.

Leverage Some individual actors can bring varied experience, widespread contacts, and a longer track record, than others and this additional input can be seen as advantageous to lever or gain greater influence.

Lobbying The attempt to influence official decisions through direct and personal communication between a lobbyist and the policymaker.

Mapping The identification, ranking and prioritisation of assets, the causes of problems and the solutions to resolve them.

Marginalisation A process by which an individual or a group is denied access to, or positions of, economic, religious and political power within a society.

Media advocacy Influences the selection, framing and debate of specific (health) topics by using the mass media.

Needs assessment A process that is used to identify the needs reported by an individual or group.

Network A structure of relationships linking social actors.

Outcome evaluation Is used to assess whether or not the programme has achieved its aims or any longer-term changes.

Partnerships Relationships with different groups or organisations based on recognition of overlapping or mutual interests and interpersonal and inter-organisational respect.

Peer education An approach in which people are supported to promote health-enhancing change among their peers.

Persuasion A process aimed at changing attitudes, beliefs or behaviours by using methods of communication to convey information, feelings or reasoning or by using one's personal or positional resources to gain leverage to change other people's behaviours or attitudes.

PhotoVoice A process by which people can identify, represent and enhance their community through a specific photographic technique.

Power (hard) The capacity of some to produce intended and foreseen effects on others.

Power (soft) The ability to obtain what one wants through indirect and long-term actions such as cooption and attraction.

Powerlessness The absence of power, whether imagined or real, and the expectancy that the behaviour of a person cannot determine the outcomes they seek.

Pressure group Collective action to change the opinions and attitudes of society and to influence the policy-making process – for example, using lobbying – but not to govern.

Process evaluation Is used to assess how the programme works once it has started and the extent to which it is being delivered effectively.

Reflexive practice Being critical about the way we use knowledge and our power to have influence over others.

Salutogenesis An approach focusing on factors that support human health and wellbeing, rather than on factors that cause disease; specifically, concerned with the relationship between health, stress and coping.

Self-help Self-help, or self-improvement, is a self-guided improvement, economically, intellectually or emotionally, often with a psychosocial basis.

Self-help group Organisation around a specific problem about which its members have a shared knowledge and interest; members are supportive of one another and often manage their own activities.

Setting A place or social context in which people engage in daily activities and in which environmental, organisational and personal factors interact to affect health and wellbeing.

Social movement A sustained and organised public effort with an ability to go beyond the influence of its participant and resource base and to maintain an ideology irrespective of membership, function and organisational structure. Social movements have 'deep social roots' and strong social networks that target those in authority to achieve their aims.

'Third sector' All not-for-profit organisations, and voluntary, community, charity and social associations.

Top-down An approach that identifies health needs in 'top' structures and then delivers these 'down' to others often at the community level.

Upstream approach The population level in which strategies address the determinants of health – for example, policy change – which relate to the conditions under which people live.

Volunteering An activity that involves spending time doing something for free that aims to benefit the environment and others, including close relatives.

References

Allsop, J., Jones, K., and Baggott, R. (2004) Health consumer groups in the UK: A new social movement. *Sociology of Health & Illness*. 26(6): 737–756.

Altogether Better (2011) York and Humberside Public Health Observatory. Accessed 23 May 2011. www.yhpho.org.uk.

Anderson, E., Shepard, M., and Salisbury, C. (2006) 'Taking off the suit': Engaging the community in primary health care decision-making. *Health Expectations*. 9: 70–80.

Antonovsky, A. (1979) *Health, stress and coping*. San Francisco: Jossey-Bass Publishers.

ASH (2012) Action on Smoking and Health. Accessed 20 December 2012. www.ash.org

Baggott, R. (2010) *Public health: Policy and politics*. 2nd edition. London: Palgrave Macmillan.

Bamberger, M., Rugh, J., and Mabry, L. (2006) *Realworld evaluation: Working under budget, time, data and political constraints*. London: Sage.

Banks, K., Eagle, N., Rotich, J., Iyoha, C., Naidoo, A., Ngolobe, B. T., Kreutz, C., Reed, R., Atwood, A., and Ekine, S. (2010). *SMS uprising: Mobile activism in Africa*. Oxford: Fahamu Books and Pambazuka Press.

Barry, M., Allegrante, J., Lamarre, M., Auld, M., and Taub, A. (2009) The Galway conference statement: International collaboration on the development of core competencies for health promotion and health education. *Global Health Promotion*. 16(2): 5–11.

Bassett, S. F., and Prapavessis, H. (2007) Home-based physical therapy intervention with adherence-enhancing strategies versus clinic-based management for patients with ankle sprains. *Physical Therapy*. 87(9): 1132–1143.

Baum, F. (2008) *The new public health*. 3rd edition. Oxford: Oxford Higher Education

Baum, F. (2011) From Norm to Eric: Avoiding lifestyle drift in Australian health policy. *Australian and New Zealand Journal of Public Health*. 35(5): 404–406.

Bell-Woodard, G., Chad, K., Labonte, R., and Martin, L. (2005) Community capacity assessment of an active living health promotion program: 'Saskatoon in Motion'. University of Saskatchewan (unpublished).

Berkman, L. (1986) Social networks, support and health: Taking the next step forward. *American Journal of Epidemiology*. 123: 559–561.

Berridge, V. (2007) Public health activism. *British Medical Journal*. 335: 1310–1312.

Bhattacharya, K., Winch, P., LeBan, K., and Tien, M. (2001) *Community health workers. Incentives and disincentives: How they affect motivation, retention and sustainability*. Published by the Basic Support for Institutionalizing

Child Survival Project (BASICS II) for the United States Agency for International Development. Arlington, Virginia.

Biddix, J. P., and Han Woo, P. (2008) Online networks of student protest: The case of the living wage campaign. *New Media and Society.* 10(6): 871–891.

Blaxter, M. (2010) *Health.* 2nd edition. Oxford: Polity Press.

Boseley, S. (2006) Herceptin costs 'put other patients at risk'. *Guardian Weekly.* December, p. 8.

Bradshaw, J. R. (1972) The concept of social need. *New Society.* 496: 640–643.

Brashers, D. E., Haas, S. M., Neidig, J. L., and Rintamaki, L. S. (2002) Social activism, self-advocacy and coping with HIV illness. *Journal of Social and Personal Relationships.* 19(1): 113–133.

Braunack-Mayer, A., and Louise, J. (2008) The ethics of community empowerment: Tensions in health promotion theory and practice. *Global Health Promotion.* 15(3): 5–8.

Brennan, L., and Binney, W. (2010) Fear, guilt and shame appeals in social marketing. *Journal of Business Research.* 63(2): 140–146.

Brown, P., and Zavestoski, S. (2004) Social movements in health: An introduction. *Sociology of Health & Illness.* 26(6): 679–694.

Brown, V. A. (1992) Health care policies, health policies or policies for health? In H. Gardner (ed.) *Health policy development, implementation and evaluation in Australia.* Melbourne: Churchill Livingstone.

Cannon, M., and Perkins, J. (2009) *Social justice handbook.* Nottingham: IVP Books.

Changing minds (2013) Whole system planning. Accessed 18 December 2013. www.changingminds.org.

Chemers, M. (1997) *An integrative theory of leadership.* Mahwah, NJ: Lawrence Erlbaum.

Christakis, N. A., and Fowler, J. H. (2007) The spread of obesity in a large social network over 32 years. *New England Journal of Medicine* 357(4): 370–379.

Chu, C., Breucker, G., Harris, N., Stitzel, A., Gan, X., Gu, X., and Dwyer, S. (2000) Health-promoting workplaces: International settings development. *Health Promotion International.* 15(2): 155–167.

Cohen-Vogel, L., and McLendon, M. (2009). New approaches to understanding federal involvement in education. In D. Plank, G. Sykes and B. Schneider (eds) *Handbook of education policy research: A handbook for the American Educational Research Association.* Mahwah, NJ: Lawrence Erlbaum.

Confederation of British Industry (CBI) (2006) *Transforming local services.* Confederation of British Industry Brief. London. July 2006.

Conway, K. (2002). Booze and beach bans: Turning the tide through community action in New Zealand. *Health Promotion International.* 17(2): 171–177.

Corcoran, N. (ed.) (2013) *Communicating health: Strategies for health promotion.* 2nd edition. London. Sage.

Craig, J., and Smyth, R. (2002) *The evidence-based practice manual for nurses.* Edinburgh: Churchill Livingstone.

Dempsey, C., Battel-Kirk, B., and Barry, M. (2011) *The CompHP core competencies framework for health promotion handbook.* Executive Agency for Health and Consumers. Paris: IUHPE.

Dixey, R., Cross, R., Foster, S., Lowcock, D., O'Neil, I., South, J., Warwick-Booth, L., White, J., and Woodall, J. (2013) *Health promotion: Global principles and practice.* Wallingford, Oxfordshire. CAB International.

Dormandy, E., Michie, S., Weinman, J., and Marteau, T. (2002) Variation in uptake of serum screening: The role of service delivery. *Prenatal Diagnosis.* 22(1): 67–69.

Draper, P. (ed.) (1991) *Health through public policy.* London: Green Print.

Dryden, W., and Feltham, C. (1993). *Brief counselling: A practical guide for beginning practitioners.* Milton Keynes: Open University Press.

Earle, L., Fozilhujaev, B., Tashbaeva, C., and Djamankulova, K. (2004) *Community development in Kazakhstan, Kyrgyzstan and Uzbekistan.* Occasional paper number 40. Oxford: INTRAC.

Edwards, M., Howard, C., and Miller, R. (2001) *Social policy, public policy: From problem to practice.* Sydney: Allen & Unwin.

Every Australian Counts (2012) accessed 17 January 2104. http://everyaustraliancounts .com.au.

Falkirk Council/HealthProm (2013) *You've got a friend in me: Befriending and volunteer scheme handbook.* London: HealthProm.

Farris Kurtz, L. (1997) *Self-help and support groups: A handbook for the practitioner.* London: Sage.

Foot, J., and Hopkins, T. (2010) *A glass half full: How an asset approach can improve community health and well-being.* London: Improvement and Development Agency (IDeA).

Forsyth, D. R. (2009) *Group dynamics.* 5th edition. Singapore: Cengage Learning.

Fox, S., and Rainie, L. (2001) Vital decisions: How internet users decide what information to trust when they or their loved ones are sick. In J. Hubley and J. Copeman (eds) (2008) *Practical health promotion.* Cambridge: Polity Press.

Freire, P. (2005) *Education for critical consciousness.* New York: Continuum Press.

Frusciante, A. K. (2007) Leadership, participatory democratic. In G. L. Andersen and K. G. Herr (eds) *Encyclopedia of activism and social justice.* London: Sage.

Gee, D. (2008) Park Scheme seeks more 'friends'. *The Christchurch Press.* Accessed 3 April 2008. www.bush.org.nz/library/934.html.

Gibbon, M., Labonte, R., and Laverack, G. (2002) Evaluating community capacity. *Health and Social Care in the Community.* 10(6):485–491.

Gillespie, D., and Melching, M. (2010) The transformative power of democracy and human rights in nonformal education: The case of Tostan. *Adult Education Quarterly.* 60(5): 477–498.

Gilmore, G. (2011) *Needs and capacity assessment for health education and health promotion.* 4th edition. Boston, MA: Jones and Bartlett Learning.

Giuntoli, G., Kinsella, K., and South, J. (2012) Evaluation of the 'Altogether Better' asset mapping in Sharrow and Firth Park, Sheffield. Leeds Metropolitan University. Institute for health and wellbeing. Leeds, UK.

Glanz, K., Rimer, B., and Viswanath, K. (eds) (2008) *Health behavior and health education: Theory, research and practice.* 4th edition. San Francisco: Jossey-Bass.

Glaser, J., and Salzberg, C. (2011) *The strategic application of information technology in health care organisations.* San Francisco: Jossey Bass.

Goodman, R. M., Speers, M. A., McLeroy, K., Fawcett, S., Kegler, M., Parker, E., Rathgeb Smith, S., Sterling, T. D., and Wallerstein, N. (1998) Identifying and defining the dimensions of community capacity to provide a basis for measurement. *Health Education and Behavior.* 25(3): 258–278.

Gottwald, M., and Goodman-Brown, J. (2012) *A guide to practical health promotion*. Maidenhead: Open University Press.

Green, L., and Kreuter, M. (2004) *Health program planning: An educational and ecological approach*. 4th edition. Maidenhead: McGraw-Hill.

Guba, E. G. (1990) *The paradigm dialog*. London: Sage.

Guba, E. G., and Lincoln, Y. S. (1989) *Fourth generation evaluation*. Newbury Park, CA: Sage.

Hager, N. (2009) Symposium on commercial sponsorship of psychiatrist education. Speech to the Royal Australian and New Zealand College of Psychiatrists Conference, Rotorua, 16 October 2009.

Hancock, T. (1993) Health, human development and the community ecosystem: Three ecological models. *Health Promotion International*. 8(1): 41–47.

Haque, N., and Eng, B. (2011) Tackling inequity through a Photovoice project on the social determinants of health: Translating Photovoice evidence to community action. *Global Health Promotion*. 18(1): 16–19.

Harris, K. (2011) Isn't all community development assets based? *The Guardian online*. Posted 23 June 2011.

Haynes, A. S., Gillespie, J. A., Derrick, G. E., Hall, W. D., Redman, S., Chapman, S., and Sturk, H. (2011) Galvanizers, guides, champions, and shields: The many ways that policymakers use public health researchers. *The Milbank Quarterly*. 89(4): 564–598.

Holder, H., Saltz, R., Grube, J., Voas, R., Gruenewald, P., and Treno, A. (1997) A community prevention trial to reduce alcohol involved accidental injury and death: Overview. *Addiction*. 92: S155–S171.

Holland, S. (2007) *Public health ethics*. Cambridge: Polity Press.

Hubley, J., and Copeman, J. (2013) *Practical health promotion*. 2nd edition. Cambridge: Polity Press.

Hull, J. (1988) Not in my neighborhood. *Time* (Time Inc). Accessed 25 January 2011. www.time.com/time/magazine/article.

Jirojwong, S. and Liamputtong, P. (eds) (2009) *Population health, communities and health promotion*. Oxford: Oxford University Press.

Johansen, E., Diop, N., Laverack, G., and Leye, E. (2013) What works and what does not: A discussion of popular approaches for the abandonment of Female Genital Mutilation. *Obstetrics and Gynaecology International*. Advance access ID 348248.

Jones, A., and Laverack, G. (2003) Building capable communities within a sustainable livelihoods approach: Experiences from Central Asia. Accessed 1 September 2003. www.livelihoods.org/lessons/CentralAsia&EasternEurope/SLLPC.

Kashefi, E., and Mort, M. (2004) Grounded citizen's juries: A tool for health activism? *Health Expectations*. 7(4): 290–302.

Kendall, S. (ed.) (1998) *Health and empowerment: Research and practice*. London: Arnold.

Klawiter, M. (2004) Breast cancer in two regimes: The impact of social movements on illness experience. *Sociology of Health & Illness*. 26(6): 845–874.

Knudsen, T. (2007) Child labor laws. In G. L. Andersen and K. G. Herr (eds) *Encyclopedia of activism and social justice*. London: Sage.

Korsching, P. F. and Borich, T. O. (1997) Facilitating cluster communities: Lessons from the Iowa experience. *Community Development Journal* 32(4): 342–353.

Kretzmann, J. P., and McKnight, J. L. (1996) *Mapping community capacity.* Evanston, IL: Institute for Policy Research, Northwestern University.

Kretzmann, J. P., and McKnight, J. L. (2007) Asset based community development. *National Civic Review.* 85(4): 23–29.

Kumpfer, K., Turner, C., Hopkins, R., and Librett, J. (1993) Leadership and team effectiveness in community coalitions for the prevention of alcohol and other drug abuse. *Health Education Research: Theory and Practice.* 8(3): 359–374.

Labonte, R. (1998) *A community development approach to health promotion: A background paper on practice tensions, strategic models and accountability requirements for health authority work on the broad determinants of health.* Edinburgh: Health Education Board for Scotland.

Labonte, R., and Laverack, G (2001) Capacity building in health promotion, part 1: For whom? And for what purpose? *Critical Public Health.* 11(2): 111–128.

Labonte, R., and Laverack, G. (2008) *Health promotion in action: From local to global empowerment.* Basingstoke: Palgrave Macmillan.

Labonte, R., and Robertson, A. (1996) Delivering the goods, showing our stuff: The case for a constructivist paradigm for health promotion and research. *Health Education Quarterly.* 23(4): 431–447.

Laverack, G. (2004) *Health promotion practice: Power and empowerment.* London. Sage.

Laverack, G. (2007) *Health promotion practice: Building empowered communities.* Maidenhead: Open University Press.

Laverack, G. (2009) *Public health: Power, empowerment and professional practice.* 2nd edition. Basingstoke: Palgrave Macmillan.

Laverack, G. (2013a) *A to Z of health promotion.* Basingstoke: Palgrave Macmillon.

Laverack, G. (2013b) *Health activism: Foundations and strategies.* London: Sage.

Laverack, G., and Whipple, A. (2010) The sirens' song of empowerment: A case study of health promotion and the New Zealand Prostitutes Collective. *Global Health Promotion.* 17(1): 33–38.

Leach, F. (1994) Expatriates as agents of cross-cultural transmission. *Compare.* 24(3): 217–231.

Lennon, R., Rentfro, R., and O'Leary, B. (2010) Social marketing and distracted driving behaviors among young adults: The effectiveness of fear appeals. *Academy of Marketing Studies Journal.* 14(2): 95–113.

Levine, D. (2008) *The art of lobbying: Building trust and selling policy* Washington, DC: CQ Press.

Libby, P. (2011) *The lobbying strategy handbook: 10 steps to advancing any cause effectively.* London: Sage.

Lin, N. (2000) Inequality in social capital. *Contemporary Sociology.* 29: 785–795.

Lindquist, E.A. (2001) Discerning policy influence: Framework for a strategic evaluation of IDRC-supported research. Accessed on 23 March 2014. www.idrc.ca/uploads/user-S/10359907080discerning_policy.pdf.

Lindström, B., and Eriksson, M. (2005) Salutogenesis. *Journal of Epidemiology and Community Health.* 59(6): 440–442.

Lindström, B., and Eriksson, M. (2010) *The hitchhiker's guide to salutogenesis: Salutogenic pathways to health promotion.* Fokhalsan Health Promotion Research Report 2. Helsinki: Fokhalsan.

Loue, S., Lloyd, L. S., and O'Shea, D. J. (2003) *Community health advocacy.* New York: Kluwer Academic/Plenum.

Lustig, S. (2012) *Advocacy strategies for health and mental health professionals: From patients to policies.* New York: Springer.

Macdowall, W., Bonell, C., and Davies, M. (2006) *Health promotion practice* (Understanding public health). Maidenhead: Open University Press.

Mackie, G. (1996) Ending foot-binding and infibulation: A convention account. *American Sociological Review.* 61(6): 999–1017.

McGrath, C. (2007) Lobbying. In G. L. Andersen and K. G. Herr (eds) *Encyclopedia of activism and social justice.* London: Sage.

McLeod, J., and McLeod, J. (2011) *A practical guide for counsellors and helping professionals.* Maidenhead: Open University Press.

MacPherson, D. W., and Gushulak, B. D. (2004) *Global migration perspectives.* Global Commission on International Migration. Geneva. Report Number 7. October 2004.

McQueen, D., and de Salazar, L. (2011) Health promotion, the Ottawa Charter and 'developing personal skills': A compact history of 25 years. *Health Promotion International.* 26 (supplement 2).

Marlatt, G. A., and Witkiewitz, K. (2010) Update on harm-reduction policy and intervention research. *Annual Review of Clinical Psychology.* 6: 591–606.

Marlatt, G. A., Larimer, M. E., and Witkiewitz, K. (2011) *Harm reduction: Pragmatic strategies for managing high-risk behaviors.* 2nd edition. New York: Guilford Press.

Marmot, M., and Wilkinson, R. (eds) (2009) *Social determinants of health.* Oxford: Oxford University Press.

Marshall, G. (1998) *A dictionary of sociology.* Oxford: Oxford University Press.

Martin, B. (2007) Activism, social and political. In G. L. Andersen and K. G. Herr (eds) *Encyclopedia of activism and social justice.* London: Sage.

Mays, N., and Pope, C. (1995) Observational methods in health care settings. *British Medical Journal.* 311: 182–184.

Ministry of Health and Pacific Island Affairs (2004) *Tupu ola moui: Pacific health chart book.* Wellington, New Zealand: Ministry of Health.

Mitchell, C., and Banks, M. (1998) *Handbook of conflict resolution: The analytical problem-solving approach.* London: Pinter.

Moana, I. (2005) Diabetes prevention in Tongan people. Project report commhlth 743. University of Auckland, Auckland. Unpublished

Monti, P. M., Colby, S. M., Barnett, N. P., Spirito, A., Rohsenow, D. J., Myers, M., Woolard, R., and Lewander, W. (1999) Brief intervention for harm reduction and alcohol practices in older adolescents in a hospital emergency department. *Journal of Counseling and Clinical Psychology.* 76(6): 989–994.

Mouy, B.,and Barr, A. (2006) The social determinants of health: is there a role for health promotion foundations? *Health Promotion Journal of Australia.*17(3):189–195.

Naidoo, J., and Wills, J. (2009) *Foundations for health promotion.* 3rd edition. Edinburgh: Baillière Tindall.

Nathanson, C., and Hopper, K. (2010) The Marmot review – social revolution by stealth. *Social Science and Medicine.* 71: 1237–1239.

National Health Service (2013) NHS values summit. www.england.nhs.uk. Accessed 18 December 2013.

Navarro, V. (2009) What we mean by social determinants of health. *Global Health Promotion.* 16(1):05–16.

Neilson, S. (2001) IDRC-supported research and its influence on public policy. knowledge utilization and public policy processes: A literature review. IDRC

Evaluation Unit. http://idrinfo.idrc.ca/archive/corpdocs/117145/litreview_e. html

NHS North West (2011) *Development of a method for asset based working*. Manchester: NHS North West and Department of Health.

Noar, S. M., and Grant-Harrington, N. (2012) *eHealth applications: Promising strategies for behaviour change*. New York: Routledge.

Nomura, S., and Ishida, T. (2003) Online communities. *Encyclopedia of community*. Accessed 5 December 2011. www.sage-ereference.com/view/community/n362.xml.

Nutbeam, D. (2000) Health literacy as a public health goal: A challenge for contemporary health education and communication strategies into the 21st century. *Health promotion international*. 15(3): 259–267.

Nutbeam, D., and Bauman, A. (2006) *Evaluation in a nutshell*. Sydney: McGraw-Hill.

Nutbeam, D,. Harris, E., and Wise, M. (2010) *Theory in a nutshell: A practical guide to health promotion theories*. 3rd edition. Maidenhead: McGraw-Hill.

Papa, M. J., Singhal, A., and Papa, W. H. (2006) *Organizing for social change: A dialectic journey of theory and praxis*. London: Sage.

Patient UK (2012). Accessed 21 May 2012. www.patient.co.uk.

Patients Association (2011). Accessed 15 December 2011. www.patients-association.com.

Pescosolido, B. A. (1991) Illness careers and network ties: A conceptual model of utilization and compliance. In G. Albrecht and J. Levy (eds) *Advances in medical sociology*. Greenwich, CT: JAI Press, pp. 161–184.

PHAC (Public Health Agency of Canada) (2013) Glossary of terms. Accessed 21 January 2013. www.phac-aspc.gc.ca/php-psp/ccph-cesp/glos-eng.php#h.

PhotoVoice (2013) Social change through photography. Accessed 5 March 2013. www.photovoice.org.

Plows, A. (2007) Strategies and tactics in social movements. In G. L. Andersen and K. G. Herr (eds) *Encyclopedia of activism and social justice*. London: Sage.

Raphael, D. (2000) The question of evidence in health promotion. *Health Promotion International*. 15(4): 355–367.

Reaves, J. (2007) Walking away from the past: How does an outsider change a culture? From the inside out says activist Molly Melching. *Chicago Tribune*. 25 November, p. 12.

Renewal.net (2008) Resolving differences – building communities and Aik saath: Conflict resolution peer group facilitators. Renewal.net case studies. Accessed 29 April 2008. www.renewal.net/Documents/RNET.

Renkert, S., and Nutbeam, D. (2001) Opportunities to improve maternal health literacy through antenatal education: An explanatory study. *Health Promotion International*. 16(4): 381–388.

Rifkin, S. B., and Pridmore, P. (2001) *Partners in planning: Information, participation and empowerment*. London: Macmillan Education.

Rissel, C. (1994) Empowerment: The holy grail of health promotion? *Health Promotion International* 9(1): 39–47.

Ritter, A., and Cameron, J. (2006) A review of the efficacy and effectiveness of harm reduction strategies for alcohol, tobacco and illicit drugs. *Drug and Alcohol Review*. 25(6): 611–624

Robertson, J., Catanzarite, J., and Hong, L. (2010) *Peer health education: Concepts and content*. San Diego, CA. University Readers.

Rohlinger, D. A., and Brown, J. (2009) Democracy, action and the internet after 9/11. *American Behavioural Scientist.* 53(1): 133–150.

Rychetnik, L., and Wise, M. (2004) Advocating evidence-based health promotion: Reflections and a way forward. *Health Promotion International.* 19(2): 247–257.

Scott, J. (2001) *Power.* Cambridge: Polity Press.

Scrambler, G. (1987) Habermas and the power of medical expertise. In G. Scrambler (ed.) *Sociological theory and medical sociology.* New York: Methuen Press.

Scriven, A. (2010) *Promoting health: A practical guide.* London:Baillière Tindall Elsevier.

Sechrest, L. E. (1997) Book review. Empowerment evaluation: knowledge and tools for self-assessment & accountability. *Environment and Behavior.* 29(3): 422–426.

Seedhouse, D. (1997) *Health promotion: Philosophy, prejudice and practice.* New York/Toronto: Wiley & Sons.

Seiter, R. H., and Gass, J. S. (2010) *Persuasion, social influence, and compliance gaining.* 4th edition. Boston, MA: Allyn & Bacon.

Seligman, M. (1990) *Learned optimism.* Toronto, ON: Pocket Books.

Smithies, J., and Webster, G. (1998) *Community involvement in health.* Aldershot: Ashgate.

South, J. (2013) Health promotion by communities and in communities: Current issues for research and practice. 7th Nordic health promotion research conference. 17–19 June 2013. Vestfold University College, Vestfold, Norway.

South, J., White, J., and Gamsu, M. (2013) *People-centred public health.* Bristol: Policy Press.

Srinivasan, L. (1993) *Tools for community participation: A manual for training trainers in participatory techniques.* New York: PROWWESS/UNDP.

Stewart, M. A., Brown, J. B., Weston, W. W., et al. (2003) *Patient centred medicine: Transforming the clinical method.* 2nd edition. Oxford: Radcliffe Medical Publications.

Syme, L. (1997) Individual vs community interventions in public health practice: Some thoughts about a new approach. *Vichealth Letter.* 2 (July): 2–9.

Taylor, L., Gowman, N., and Quigley, K. (2003) *Evaluating health impact assessment.* London: Health Development Agency.

Tengland, P. (2007) Empowerment: A goal or a means for health promotion? *Medicine, Health Care and Philosophy.* 10: 197–207.

Tengland, P. (2013) Behavior change or empowerment: On the ethics of health promotion goals. *Health Care Analysis.* 8 October 2013.

Tones, K., and Tilford, S. (2001) *Health education: Effectiveness, efficiency and equity.* 3rd edition. London: Nelson Thornes.

UNICEF (2001) *Beyond child labour: Affirming rights.* New York: UNICEF.

UNICEF (2013) *Peer education.* Accessed 21 January 2013. www.unicef.org/lifeskills/index_12078.html.

United Way (2012) *Building strong neighbourhoods: Neighbourhoods report.* Toronto, ON: United Way.

Van Ryn, M., and Heany, C. (1992) What's the use of theory? *Health Education Quarterly.* 19(3): 315–330.

Volunteering England (2012) *What is volunteering?* Accessed 5 January 2014. www.volunteering.org.uk.

Wagenaar, A., Murray, D., and Toomey, T. (2000). Communities moblilizing for change on alcohol: Effects of a randomized trial on arrests and traffic crashes. *Addiction.* 95: 209–217.

Walker, K., MacBride, A., and Vachon, M. (1977) Social support networks and the crisis of bereavement. *Social Science and Medicine.* 11: 35–41.

Wallack, L. M., Dorfman, L., Jernigan, D., and Makani, T. (1993) *Media advocacy and public health.* London: Sage.

Wallerstein, N. (2006) *What is the evidence on effectiveness of empowerment to improve health?* Health Evidence Network report. Copenhagen: WHO Regional Office for Europe.

Wallerstein, N., and Bernstein, E. (1988) Empowerment education: Freire's ideas adapted to health education. *Health Education Quarterly.* 15(4): 379–394.

Walt, G. (1994) *Health policy: An introduction to process and power.* London: Zed Books.

Weatherburn, D. (2009) Dilemmas in harm minimization. *Addiction.* 104(3): 335–339.

Werner, D. (1988) Empowerment and health: Contact. *Christian Medical Commission.* 102: 1–9.

Wharf-Higgins, J., Naylor, P. J., Day, M. (2007) Seed funding for health promotion: Sowing sustainability or scepticism? *Community Development Journal.* Advance access 31 January 2007: 1–12.

Wilkinson, R. G. (ed.) (2003) *Social determinants of health: The solid facts.* 2nd edition. Copenhagen: WHO Regional Office for Europe.

Winfield, M. (2013) *The essential volunteer handbook.* Victoria, BC: Friesen Press.

Wood, S., Sawyer, R., and Simpson-Hebert, M. (1998) *PHAST step-by-step-guide.* Geneva: WHO.

World Health Organization (1986) *Ottawa charter for health promotion.* Geneva: WHO.

World Health Organization (1988) Conference statement: The Adelaide recommendations. Accessed 23 March 2014. www.who.int/healthpromotion/conferences/previous/adelaide/en/index6.html.

World Health Organization (1991) *Sundsvall statement on supportive environments for health.* Geneva: WHO.

World Health Organization (1997) *The Jakarta declaration on leading health promotion into the 21st century.* Geneva: WHO.

World Health Organization (1998) *The health promotion glossary.* Geneva: WHO.

World Health Organization (2000) *Mexico global conference for health promotion.* Geneva: WHO.

World Health Organization (2005) *The Bangkok charter for health promotion in a globalized world.* 6th Global Conference on Health Promotion. Geneva: WHO.

World Health Organization (2007) *Community health workers: What do we know about them?* Geneva: WHO.

World Health Organization (2008) *Closing the gap in a generation.* Commission on Social Determinants of Health. Final Report. Geneva: WHO.

World Health Organization (2009) *The Nairobi 7th global conference on health promotion.* Geneva: WHO.

World Health Organization (2013) *The 8th global conference on health promotion.* Helsinki statement on Health in All Policies. Geneva: WHO.

World Health Organization (2014) *Health in All Policies (HiAP): Framework for country action*. Geneva: WHO.

Wright, E. R. (1997) The impact of organizational factors on mental health professionals' involvement with families. *Psychiatric Services*. 48: 921–927.

Wright, J. (2001) Assessing health needs. In D. Pencheon, J. A. Muir Gray, C. Guest, and D. Melzer (eds) *Oxford handbook of public health practice*. Oxford: Oxford University Press, pp. 38–47.

Wrong, D. H. (1988) Power. Its Forms, Bases and Uses. Chicago, USA. The University of Chicago Press.

Young, L., and Everitt, J. (2004) *Advocacy groups*. Vancouver: University of British Columbia Press.

Zakus, J. D. L., and Lysack, C. L. (1998) Revisiting community participation. *Health Policy and Planning*. 13(1): 1–12.

Index

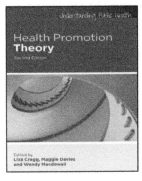

HEALTH PROMOTION THEORY
Second Edition

Liza Cragg, Maggie Davies and Wendy
Macdowall

9780335263202 (Paperback)
October 2013

eBook also available

Part of the *Understanding Public Health* series, this book offers students and
practitioners an accessible exploration of the origins and development of health
promotion. It highlights the philosophical, ethical and political debates that influence
health promotion today while also explaining the theories, frameworks and
methodologies that help us understand public health problems and develop effective
health promotion responses.

Key features:

- Offers more in-depth coverage of key determinants of health and how these
  interact with health promotion
- Revised structure to allow more depth of coverage of health promotion theory
- Updated material and case examples that reflect contemporary health
  promotion challenges

www.openup.co.uk
OPEN UNIVERSITY PRESS
McGraw - Hill Education

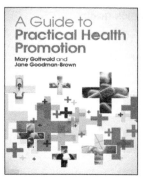

A GUIDE TO PRACTICAL HEALTH PROMOTION

Mary Gottwald and Jane Goodman-Brown

9780335244591 (Paperback)
August 2012

eBook also available

Do you have difficulties deciding which health promotion activities facilitate behavioural change?

This accessible book focuses on the practical activity of health promotion and shows students and practitioners how to actually apply health promotion in practice. The book uses case scenarios to explore how health promotion activities can empower individuals to make decisions that change their health related behaviour

Key features:

- Each chapter uses classic case studies in health promotion
- Includes lists, key points and other succinct tools to give the reader guidance
- Contains activities and specific tasks that can be used in practice

www.openup.co.uk
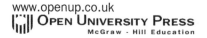 OPEN UNIVERSITY PRESS
McGraw - Hill Education

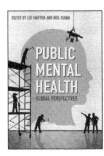

PUBLIC MENTAL HEALTH
GLOBAL PERSPECTIVES

Lee Knifton and Neil Quinn (Eds)

2013
9780335244898 (Paperback)

eBook also available

Mental health is a fundamental public health priority, and this stimulating and comprehensive book brings together all of the key issues to offer an overview for students and practitioners alike. Written by a team of leading international experts, the book summarizes the evidence base and asks the key questions at the heart of a range of topics from community development to public mental health in schools and recovery and well-being.

The book includes:

- **Mini toolkits** at the end of each chapter that include tips for effective practice, reflection points and questions to consider
- **Case studies** exploring real world examples of public mental health in action
- **Discussion** and opinion encouraging readers to question and debate the issues at the core of public mental health policy

The book also includes a chapter written by Kate E. Pickett and Richard G. Wilkinson, authors of the bestselling book *The Spirit Level*.

Public Mental Health: Global Perspectives is an invaluable tool to give readers the confidence to develop effective mental health tools and programs that will improve public mental health.

www.openup.co.uk
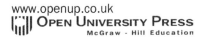
OPEN UNIVERSITY PRESS
McGraw - Hill Education

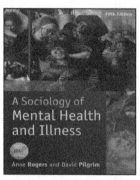

**A SOCIOLOGY OF MENTAL HEALTH
AND ILLNESS**
Fifth Edition

Anne Rogers and David Pilgrim

9780335262762 (Paperback)
May 2014

eBook also available

How do we understand mental health problems in their social context?
A former BMA Medical Book of the Year award winner, this book provides a
sociological analysis of major areas of mental health and illness. The book
considers contemporary and historical aspects of sociology, social psychiatry,
policy and therapeutic law to help students develop an in-depth and critical approach
to this complex subject.

Key features:

- Brand new chapter on prisons, criminal justice and mental health
- Expanded coverage of stigma, class and social networks
- Updated material on the Mental Capacity Act, Mental Health Act and the
  Deprivation of Liberty

www.openup.co.uk
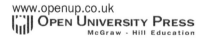

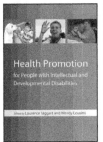

HEALTH PROMOTION FOR PEOPLE WITH INTELLECTUAL AND DEVELOPMENTAL DISABILITIES

Laurence Taggart and Wendy Cousins (Eds)

January 2014
9780335246946 (Paperback)

eBook also available

People with learning disabilities are affected by significantly more health problems than the general population and are much more likely to have significant health risks. Yet evidence suggests they are not receiving the same level of health education and health promotion opportunities as other members of society.

This important, interdisciplinary book is aimed at increasing professional awareness = of the importance of health promotion activities for people with intellectual and developmental disabilities. Written by an international board of experts, it is a thorough and comprehensive guide for students, professionals and carers.

The book considers a variety of challenges faced by those with intellectual disabilities, from physical illnesses such as diabetes, epilepsy and sexual health issues, through to issues such as addiction, mental health and ageing.

www.openup.co.uk
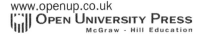
OPEN UNIVERSITY PRESS
McGraw - Hill Education